A Healthy Spirit
Surviving Cancer Christian style

Author: Lo Mallory R.D., MPH

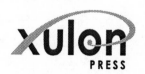

A Healthy Spirit
by Lo Mallory R.D., MPH

Printed in the United States of America

ISBN 1-60034-165-9

BIBLE REFERENCES:

God's Word
> The Scripture readings designated by (God's Word) have been taken from GOD'S WORD, copyright © 1995 by God's Word to the Nations Bible Society. All rights reserved. Used by permission.

MSG
> The Message, Colorado Springs: Navpress, 1993

NIV
> Scripture quotations taken from the HOLY BIBLE, NEW INTERNATIONAL VERSION NIV Copyright 1973, 1978, 1984 by International Bible Society. Zondervan Publishing. All rights reserved. "NIV" and "New International Version" are registered trademarks of International Bible Society.

TEV
> Today's English Version. New York: American Bible Society. 1992

TLB
The Living Bible. Wheaton, IL: Tyndale House Publishers, 1971

Illustrations are courtesy of DaySpring Cards, Inc. by written permission.

Photo in text courtesy of Renee R. Joy

www.xulonpress.com

DEDICATION

To my daughters, Katie and Renee
And
My nieces, Andrea and Alicia

Also to the prayer supporters and friends who never
stopped nurturing my Spirit and kept it healthy all
through my health crisis and today. BLESS YOU!

ACKNOWLEDGMENT

To Marie E. Nelson, John W. James, Lynn Mears and Jodie McClure I will be forever grateful for their editing and copyediting talents delivered with love, insights and encouragement.

CONTENTS

INTRODUCTION

B eing a two-year breast cancer survivor, I have been richly blessed to write this book. I have found there is no match for loving, Christian support in a crisis. My spirit was nurtured and cared for, keeping it both healthy and happy, while my unhealthy body tended to its physical needs.

If you are currently facing a health crisis, may some ideas in this book both comfort and give your spirit hope. For those who are caregivers, I offer insight into the dimensions of a care-receiver's spiritual and emotional needs.

This is neither my story nor my journal…but in looking back I realized what helped me was scripture providing the cornerstone for my strength and courage while a cancer patient. No other book, intervention or other support strategy supported me as securely as affirmations of the Christian faith. God's promises for each of us are readily available and recorded in the Bible. Passages I've selected to share with you meant a great deal to me and gave me strength. I hope your heart is open to allowing the scripture to support and guide you too.

A tactic for surviving a major illness is to hold a big picture view allowing us to understand each step of the path to recovery while maintaining the vision of striving for a positive outcome of physical and spiritual health. I agree with Maya Angelou who said, "I've learned that no matter what happens, or how bad it seems today, life does go on, and it will be better tomorrow."

A major illness is a formidable challenge. Cling to all the positive energy available while dodging the negative energy that leads to fear, stress and anxiety. Dwelling on doubts, insecurities and all that is negative lessens your positive attitude and must be recognized and put behind you. Our society and communication technologies load us with negative energy daily. In just one news broadcast, we are barraged with murders, terrorists, car accidents, reports of child abuse and on and on. Maybe you don't need to know every detail. One click of the remote and you can skip the negative energy input from media.

ON TO VICTORY

One of the media negatives I dispatched with early on was the newspaper. In the obituary section of every major newspaper, you can find this statement daily: ".. after a long and courageous battle with cancer (ALS, etc,)..." This will impact anyone with a diagnosis to match. I have a huge issue with the "battle" analogy because it implies that the deceased clearly LOST a battle. We have read those words so many times we start to believe that we are in a losing battle right from the beginning. Just talking about a battle brings up images of war, dying and wounded soldiers, blasts, fire, carnage, crying, hate, fear and bloodshed. To *battle* a disease, then, floods us in negative images and wastes energy while we endlessly worry about defeat. No battle is ever won if defeat is assumed from the start.

It is not about winning or losing the battle – it's about living your life. Join me in leaving all the negatives of a battle behind and focusing only on the positive. Like "victory" – now that is one word from a battle that energizes me.

The Bible has many references to battles, war, armies and soldiers. Soldiers march. Universally, all little kids love to march. A fond memory of my early Sunday School days in the basement of the old church was the music time before our classes met. We would sing the song the leader chose and then the piano player took a couple of requests. Every week we belted out "Onward, Christian Soldiers" while marching in place. When I was ten years old, a new, larger church was built a mile away. The day it was dedicated, the whole Sunday School marched to the new church carrying banners and singing our favorite, "Onward, Christian Soldiers." It was a positive victory march. This image (among others) lifted my spirit and recharged my batteries. This scripture provides transitioning for our thinking in terms of a win-lose battle to where we can go to find strength and victory:

"You won't (succeed) by might or by power, but by my Spirit, says the Lord of Armies."
Zechariah 4:6b (God's Word)

In choosing to focus on His Spirit, on the victory of His power, I was given the inner strength for each day, every step of the way. If you have a disease, you are a "survivor" from the minute that the diagnosis is official. So, from one survivor to another, let me help you look at ways to maximize the positive and keep the negative suppressed. Accept God's gift of grace and allow the Holy Spirit to gently guide and support your spirit whether it is living in a healthy or unhealthy body. It will make all the difference.

KAPOWEE!!!!

KAPOWEE!! Hit right square between the eyes. Being zapped by a stun gun or feeling a shock wave charge through our whole body barely describes the natural response we have to those three words, "You have cancer." Like everyone else, I knew cancer, car accidents and all other possible tragedies happen to someone else, not me.

Self-preservation being a driving force for everyone, the challenge begins with trying to focus on or fully comprehend what your ears heard. A reliable source, typically a physician, informs you that you have a serious illness, and particularly one that does not come with a guarantee for a cure, easily sparks disbelief. In Minnesota, we refer to this as a "deer in the headlights moment." Somehow, even knowledge that risk factors were present does not override the disbelief factor. Why wouldn't our intellect try to soften the blow?

Everyone deals with mini crisis situations fairly regularly. There are those who barely recognize a mini crisis as a problem and those who "fly off the handle." Whatever your orientation or experience, a minor crisis just does not compare nor prepare you for a major crisis. Even endless problem solving at your job does not prepare you for a health crisis.

We move on to asking a round of questions to verify that any tests done were actually ours and not results for someone else waiting in the exam room next door. Physicians will tie the symptoms to test results or other medical data that were the basis for the diagnosis. Assured no mistake has been made, the mind may feel cheated.

Anger may be a normal feeling initially, but try not to let it push you into a victim mentality. Anger quickly generates negative energy and may open the door for feeling a need to blame someone. The blame will show itself by being critical of the people trying to help you. If resentment is brewing under the surface, negative feelings will flourish, drag you down and fuel anxiety. Many of us need an opportunity to vent in order to let the anger go. By supporting us rather than feeling sorry for us, family and friends will lead us away from 'victim' thinking.

Quite often with only partially moving from disbelief status, *denial* returns to nudge the self-preservation mode again. We all are able to look back and remember times when we had hoped denial would rescue us from something or from some event that was unpleasant to us. Denial stays in the foreground of our thoughts as long as it is fed by our fears. KAPOWEE – the bad news comes down all at once and is incredibly overwhelming. A good place to turn is Psalm 56 and read first hand about trusting in God in this time of fear. Jesus knows we will experience fears and he directs us on how to deal with fear:

"Jesus said, Don't be afraid; just believe." Mark 5:36 NIV

In the aftermath of any traumatic event, we all progress thru the denial phase at different rates. However what seems true for most people is that our denial is rarely a full 100% or it would not cause us to be uncomfortable. If only a minute 1% of reality is on the conscious level, there is still an inner need to try to cope with the situation and move beyond denial. Perhaps it's the need to feel in control. A cancer diagnosis will make you feel like all of the control in your life has been taken away. Uncertainty and fear begin to surface as you recognize this crisis is NOT happening to someone else, but to you. At a very elemental level, fear of moving beyond denial means reality will have to be addressed – the crisis has to be acknowledged. Truly, these are the icy cold fingers of fear gripping you.

For the Christian, there is rescue from this mental anguish.

"... I am the Lord your God – and I say to you, Don't be afraid; I am here to help you." Isaiah 41:13 TLB

"....my heart shall know no fear! I am confident that God will save me." Psalms 27:3 TLB

Fear is a very real human emotion and it can be intense. To allow yourself to slip by the emotion of fear in a crisis would not be normal. As we come to grips with the fear, the denial of reality can start to fade. As denial fades, thoughts will return to wanting to regain control of our lives, bodies and the situation/crisis. I sought out God's promises for how I would get through my crisis.

"The Lord himself goes before you and will be with you...." Deuteronomy 31:8 NIV

If there was a time in your life that you faced a huge challenge, try to remember what and who helped. In what way did you seek out resources to regain personal security and a sense of comfort? At the same time, how did you separate yourself from those who were not helpful or drained you by burdening you with negative energy? Give yourself permission to unload the negatives. When I was being bombarded with a diagnosis and all its implications, the loss of control, denial and fears dominated my feelings and I just wanted to be rescued and whisked off to a safe place.

"I went to the Lord for help, He answered me and rescued me from all my fears." Psalm 34:4 (God's Word)

SEEKING SAFETY

No other descriptive word but *"overwhelming"* describes the inner conflict of sorting out the fear, denial and run-and-hide feelings. A friend of mine jokes that when things get too tough he will jump the next ice floe and float out into the ocean. Hiding from a problem doesn't make it go away, as no solution or resolution can be reached. To hide or not confront the crisis leaves you feeling out of control and a mere victim of circumstance. If you run from the crisis, courage will elude you and you will not grow. What is to be gained from being unprepared for the life changes that will happen?

"A person's fear sets a trap (for him), but one who trusts the Lord is safe." Proverbs 29:25 (God's Word)

"I have commanded you, 'Be strong and courageous! Don't tremble or be terrified, because the Lord your God is with you wherever you go." Joshua 1:9 (God's Word)

As I struggled with my cancer, I knew I didn't want to hide, but I also felt the magnitude of the overwhelming diagnosis in front of me. I sought to regain some control, only in the context of it being a safe move. God promises so much safety and protection in the scriptures that a tremendous amount of reassurance flowed around me, enabling me to take the first tiny steps away from denial and basic fear. When absolutely nothing was certain in my life, the scriptures kept me grounded. Feeling no strength of my own, I just hung on tightly to:

"God is our refuge and strength, an ever-present help in times of trouble." Psalm 46:1 (God's Word)

"I saw God. The God who can't sit still when the storm is too strong. The God who lets me get frightened enough to need him and then comes close enough for me to see him. The God who uses my storms as his path to come to me. I saw God. It took a storm for me to see him. But I saw him." Lucado's <u>Eye of the Storm</u> pg. 182.

"In their distress they cried out to the Lord. He rescued them from their troubles." Psalm 107:6 (God's Word)

One of Max Lucado's favorite stories must be from Matthew 14. It is the classic passage wherein Jesus walks on water and saves Peter from drowning in his boat in a storm because he walks to Jesus on the water. For Peter to step out onto a stormy sea, it had to be a move of desperation, yet loaded with trust. Having a major illness is very much like being in the eye of a storm. It's in the hour of our deepest need that we come begging for help, hoping our faith will be enough. "Faith is not born at the negotiating table where we barter our gifts in exchange for God's goodness. Faith is not an award given to the most learned. It's not a prize given to the most disciplined. It's not a title bequeathed to the most religious. Faith is a desperate dive out of the sinking boat of human effort and a prayer that God will be there to pull us out of the water." Lucado pg. 203.

It is God's gift of grace that will save us and keep us on His path. During the difficult times of fighting a disease, the very stormy times, it is your faith that will keep you strong and assure you your life has a purpose. In the story, Peter let his doubts and fears surface a second time. Jesus reached for him again and pulled him to safety. I lost count of how many times I made that frantic grab for safety.

"You, Lord, are the light that keeps me safe. I am not afraid of anyone. You protect me, and I have no fears.
In times of trouble, you will protect me. You will hide me in your tent and keep me safe on top of a mighty rock." Psalm 27: 1,5 NIV

In the passage below, it was easy for me to interpret the raging water as the overwhelming feeling. My mind was screaming to just get me out!

"He reached down from high above and took hold of me. He pulled me out of the raging water." Psalm 18:16 (God's Word)

In Mark 6: 45-51, Jesus walks on water to reach the boat where the disciples were rowing frantically in the heavy winds. When Jesus enters the boat, the wind calms down to the disciples amazement. Much of our life is spent rowing. "There are moments of glamour, days of celebration. We have our share of feasts, but we also have our share of baloney sandwiches. And to have the first we must endure the second. When you can't see God, trust him." Lucado's Gentle Thunder pg. 30.

"So, do not fear, for I (God) am with you;.." Isaiah 41:10 NIV

I found it true that I had to gather up the courage to move away from my fears, from any hiding place I thought I had, and make the first move to feeling somewhat back in control. I went in search of information so I could be an active participant in the decisions to be made. Having some understanding helped me cope and quieted some of my fears. Knowledge is power and I charged after a crash course. I wanted both a hands-on guide of the basics and internet access to all the latest research news.

First, given to me as a gift from the Susan G. Komen Breast Cancer Foundation, Minnesota Affiliate, was their A Handbook of Hope and Healing 2003-2004. It was the perfect resource covering all the important topics in understandable terminology. Now dated, I highly recommend securing a similar current guide from a reliable source. Be wary of information that is really selling a product or cure as its main objective. You want basic, good information about the type of cancer you have and an overview of treatment options.

Second, use your favorite search engine on the internet and uncover a wealth of information about the diagnosis you have. It's a tremendous resource, but I caution you again to stick with the reliable sources of information such as The American Cancer Society at www.cancer.org for all cancers, or the website www.breastcancer.org. You are not looking for product sales or opinions as much as factual data to help you feel you have the knowledge to understand the diagnosis. I found the website above very helpful for having a concise description that I could send by e-mail to my daughters. They were then able to explore more on the websites for their own information. They found some details their overwhelmed mother forgot to tell them. Once involved in the research, they sent me the information they found – it helped all of us.

If you are a care-giver or supporter, offering to do a little research is a nice gift, especially for those who do not easily use the internet or have no computer handy. It is a time for the basics. 'More than needed to know' interesting facts should be kept for later. How much information desired is individual – listen to the request and clarify if in doubt. A few evenings on the internet hardly compares to the training of an oncologist. But basic knowledge quiets fears and gives you some control of your life again. I was able to venture out of my hiding place and inch along beyond the initial shock.

And what was waiting for me? Decisions – huge decisions on how to best manage my health crisis.

WHY ME?

"Life brings sorrows and joys alike, it is what a man does with them – not what they do to him – that is the test of his mettle."
Teddy Roosevelt

Why me? Who has ever been given the diagnosis of a serious illness and not asked that straightforward question? I encourage you to completely clear your mind and both accept and celebrate that there is no one else like you. You are totally unique, and while others have had the same disease, you are still not the same as everyone or anyone else. At the very basic level of genetics, no one will match you 100%. Add all the other factors like tolerance to pain, medical history, effects of stress, smoking and eating habits, environmental influences, sensitivity to medications, the list goes on and on. We can all certainly learn from others who have had similar experiences – just do not lose sight of your own uniqueness.

"The rain falls on the just and the unjust." Hopi (Native American)

When it comes to cancer, I doubt any American over the age of 16 does not know of at least one person who has died from cancer and at least one person who is a survivor. It's beneficial to change one's mindset from "why me", as quick as possible, to planning on being a survivor. Discouragement and temptation to embrace self-pity is the "why me" gone too far. Trying to prove to yourself and others that you did not really have the risk factors, and therefore should not have the diagnosis, will do little but feed into negative energy and invite the negatives to overshadow the positives.

Comparing our lives with others is a human tendency. Should we start to question the justice of God or attempt to rationalize our devotion, we start to walk a fine line. By making our human understanding of justice and fairness a condition for our faith in God, we have no faith at all. Try to let the 'Why me?' go. The question itself breeds resentment and anger. If successful in hanging onto resentment, bitterness will be your companion. It locks in negative energy. We can learn from resentment and then move on.

"To worry yourself to death with resentment would be a foolish, senseless thing to do." Job 5:2 TEV

FEAR

Many people will be driven by basic fear of the disease. The word 'cancer' never elicits a positive feeling or smile to anyone's face. If anything, it throws us all into an 'on guard' position, dread or fear. But, if we allow ourselves to be driven by fear or controlled by this emotion, we can miss opportunities as our fears will hold us back. Playing it safe, avoiding risks, maintaining status quo or reverting back to denial all hold you back. Grasp your faith and establish trust – it's the way out of fear and will turn your energy from negative to positive.

"….if you do not stand firm in your faith, you will not stand at all." Isaiah 7:9 NIV

Grasping your faith will help you bring the health crisis into perspective and smooth off the rough edges. Stu Weber in his book Spirit Warriors says it as eloquently as anyone could, "When the going gets tough, the tough run straight to God!" Weber, pg. 229. In running to God, the wondering how it all happened is less important and our trust shifts to God to be our guide, to direct our spirits and secure our future.

"Call on me in times of trouble. I will rescue you, and you will honor me." Psalm 50:15 (God's Word)

Part of wondering 'why me?' may involve blaming others or external circumstances such as pesticides, radiation exposure, etc. for our health condition. Too much effort and time wallowing in these negative thoughts of being a victim is guaranteed to bring you down. The quicker we accept we cannot change the past, and both want and need to move on, will help. Trust in God to point you in the right direction by being open and by paying attention. Make the effort to direct your thoughts toward the outcome you desire and request God's grace to come to you for guidance and help.

You are a unique individual and God's plan for you is unique and custom made just for you. Be wary of putting too much trust in someone else's view of what you should do. In some ways, others' views may prevent you from receiving grace-inspired insights. The Lord is readily available to all of us with a plan just for you – your very own.

Input from others has its place as long as it does not deter us from our own inner spiritual guidance. The language of grace has been described as intuition. We need only to listen to this intuition that gained its wisdom from your own spirit. We have all experienced situations when the timing seemed all wrong, yet our intuition convinced us to move ahead and we felt guidance. Being in touch with our intuition opens the door for God's grace to guide us in the direction God planned for us to go.

"Turn all your anxiety over to God because he cares for you." 1 Peter 5:7 (God's Word)

I totally accept that I was guided by God to land in the medical offices of the surgeon, oncologist and a number of other medical team staff that I was referred to for treatment of cancer. The need to establish trust with those you feel are competent to manage your uniqueness if not your very life, is essential. At the same time, other medical practitioners could have managed my treatment plan and yet, I knew I was where I was supposed to be for God's plan for me to unfold as it did.

When I was diagnosed with cancer, I was fortunate to be living in a large metropolitan area – the Twin Cities in Minnesota. I had the luxury of being in a competitive health care market and with health insurance that allowed me coverage with the majority of providers. This gave me choices and opportunities to select physicians, hospitals for surgery and the option to explore a variety of support services for cancer patients. Marge was in treatment at the same time I was and at the same clinics. Her home was 80 miles north of the Twin Cities which was a distance burden. She stayed with an old friend on a bed and breakfast arrangement Monday through Thursday nights and went home on weekends. It was a practical gift of support and priceless to Marge.

MEDICAL SUPPORT TEAM

The basic human need to feel safe in a medical situation means you must completely trust those who hold your life and death in their hands. It is a huge and very stressful task to meet with a new physician and to promptly feel comfortable. The bottom line is we need to feel like a person with a unique illness. We seek treatment which has worked for others and at the same time we want treatment modified to our individual characteristics. Some have relayed to me they felt they were a mere medical chart number and not really a person. Trust is very hard to establish in such a situation. If you cannot feel a level of trust, seek a second opinion and a third if necessary. Not all personalities go together harmoniously. For major illnesses, it can be a long haul with many appointments – try to get comfortable on the front end and skip the stress later. Walking through the door with the 'Oncology Clinic" sign above it for the first time brought a full dose of reality for my husband and me.

"He will have no fear of bad news; his heart is steadfast, trusting in the Lord." Psalm 112:7 NIV

Well-meaning friends and family often push a newly diagnosed person to a physician they know, or more often to one they have heard about through another person. The intention is good, but a word of caution. The decision is yours alone as it's your trust, your comfort and your choice. Give yourself at least a day to think through major decisions. In prayer, ask God for the wisdom to make the right choices. Seek the guidance of the Holy Spirit.

"If any of you lacks wisdom, he should ask God, who gives generously to all without finding fault, and it will be given to him." James 1:5 NIV

I cannot fully describe the stress I felt during those long 24 hours when trying to make a decision. In comparing notes with other friends with cancer, I know we all feel this. I found those of us who prayed for the guidance and wisdom to make the right choices felt peace of mind gently overcome us. Our prayers were answered and the anxiety of indecision left us. I felt changed or touched by God so that I could see my situation and the path I was intended to follow. I then went forward with more confidence and others commented on my positive attitude. God had provided the peace that became visible to others.

"Peace I (Jesus) leave with you; my peace I give you. I do not give to you as the world gives. Do not let your hearts be troubled and do not be afraid." John 14:27 NIV

Get a handle on the self-pity; recognize any form of discouragement coming your way and deal with it or the source. You don't have to let someone else take you down. I was advised to NOT communicate with someone who pushed my buttons and tender balance to the edge. This person meant well no doubt, but lacked the vision to realize the damage being done. Caller ID – what a great invention.

NO RIGHT ANSWER

Before we leave this topic, a suggestion for caregivers: remember to listen. When someone has just been diagnosed with a major illness and they are asking 'Why me?' refrain from answering. There is absolutely NO right answer. We need someone to listen, and we may need just to vent. We know there's no right answer. For caregivers and friends, know that the person staring the crisis in the face is *very, very* sensitive, tender, and emotionally fragile. Choose words carefully and help your loved one or friend by leading into positive encouragement. Talk about survivors and certainly not the person you knew who had the same diagnosis and died. I would not mention this if it hadn't happened to me.

It almost sounds selfish, but I am sure I was testing the waters for who would support me. Who could I lean on and know they wouldn't be judgmental and/or tell me I was foolish to be so scared? Conflicting opinions or basic disagreements with those close to me would certainly complicate the already difficult decision process. At the same time, I was working to secure my physicians. I was honestly surprised that I felt so much trust in all my physicians on the first visit. I was secure in my choices and knew I would not seek second opinions. However, my peace of mind was interrupted by others who were insistent I check out other doctors, other clinics, etc. Naturally, each one had a different clinic in mind and each gave me names and phone numbers. I guess I was lucky none of them kidnapped me and dragged me into their choice. For each of these well-meaning people, after they heard I had found my physician and was not interested in a second opinion, they still went ahead with their advice. Not only did they not listen but it was inferred my choice was incorrect. At no other time in my life had I been so vulnerable to criticism or what under my intense stress I perceived to be criticism.

The last position a person who is seeking support wants to be put in is a defensive position. If for no other reason, limited sleep and exhaustion just do not allow it. Decisions take huge amounts of mental and physical energy. One caring friend, Paula, who is a cancer survivor, offered on a greeting card to give me the name and number of her doctor should I want them. I know Paula was not offended when I didn't call to get the number.

I did call Paula, however, to thank her and also to tell her I had found a doctor. She responded by affirming my decision and was happy for me to be spared a long search. Paula also taught me the valuable lesson that while many people get diagnosed with breast cancer, we are all individuals and everyone is different. It's our uniqueness that makes us comfortable with trusting one doctor and not another. Breast cancer is a general name and tells us little of the specifics or exact type of the disease. We each uniquely respond to treatments. Now that I am a survivor too, Paula has added two words, "Everyone is so different, aren't they?" I agree.

Please support those who need you where they are. Support is listening to why they chose the doctor they did. Affirming their trust and comfort level is the most important part of the decision. Anyone with a mountain of stress needs the support of a listener and someone to affirm they are doing the right thing. Listen, as sometimes the right thing is to get a second or third opinion. This listening and affirming continues in being supportive of whatever choice is made for treatment of the disease. Remember whose choice it is, even when the choice is to do nothing to stop the disease. Just listen and know some questions really have no answers. Medical questions should be directed back to the medical support team.

GOING TO THE DOGS

I regret I have not been able to get my mixed breed dog, known to friends and family as the '"Love Dog," to verbally express her experiences in life. She was the one being I could trust unconditionally to listen to my concerns and hear me out on the big questions of my crisis. Love Dog offered no advice. She was delighted to have a frequent nap companion. Pets are marvelous therapy. We can all learn from the many programs helping young children to read by practicing their reading to a dog. Dogs never laugh at mistakes, never criticize or try to correct the reader. They simply listen. Confidence can build and security is felt with that exchange. We will look later at using pets for home therapy.

Answered prayers were always a blessing and clearly felt right. Having dear friends who were praying for me, I specifically asked them to pray that my physicians would have the skills and expertise to take care of me and I receive the wisdom to make the right decisions.

The anxiety in the pre-decisions stage went away. LOVE THAT PEACE OF MIND!!

"He alone is my Rock, my rescuer, defense and fortress – why then should I be tense with fear when troubles come?"
Psalm 62:6 TLB

GOD'S PLAN

I knew early on that God had a plan for me and for my life. The first book I picked up (or was led to choose) once I had recovered enough to venture back into shopping in stores again was The Purpose Driven Life by Rick Warren. This book explains so well the concept of God's plan. I encourage you to read his book, particularly Chapter 2 titled "You Are Not an Accident."

God's plans, purposes and priorities resist our attempts to reduce them to an orderly outline. We desire the logical or to look for the right icon key to spell it out for us. If only we could push the "help" or F1 key. Quite possibly we are just reacting to the reality that our plan for our own life has changed. Before being diagnosed with cancer, I was happily bouncing along through life without a clue. After a couple careers in the medical business field, it came as a shock that I, overnight, had become the one labeled 'the patient'. If you watch enough sci-fi, you can relate to walking through a swirling colored liquid wall from the life you knew, to being on the other side as the patient. With a newfound cancer, you are referred to a specialist and leave behind the physician who knows you medically and personally. Still in the shock and denial phase, we meet the specialist who sees you "as you are" that day and has no idea who you were on the other side of the liquid wall prior to you falling through the wall. One thing the new doctor does know, for sure, is that no one had it as his or her personal plan in life to be there. Changes on top of changes are the new norm.

I used to write a business plan annually for my employer. There it was, all laid out for the year, including the budget. Following the business plan with as minimal modifications equaled success and possibly a raise in a good year. We are all managers on the home front too. Without a plan in place, how would groceries get in the kitchen, children bussed to sports or music lessons, laundry done, dental appointments, etc.? We are used to managing our own affairs and doing so with some plan in place. It certainly was not my plan to enter into this major change in health status or life changing experience.

There's little doubt a challenge lies ahead. The hustle and bustle of daily life will slow, as activities and the plans of the normal, healthy lifestyle get put on hold while you deal with your health challenge. It's been referred to as 'active waiting', to make adjustments from the daily usual life to giving attention to the health crisis. It's through the slowing down, listening and watching for the signs that God will provide, that we can move into accepting that God's plan for each of us is now in place and has been, for a long time. Change is not easy, yet we only need to follow.

Whether you are the organized type or happy in disorganization, believing God has a plan exclusively for you is security. To know the plan is there also means accepting it. We were not involved in writing the outline nor designing it. We do not KNOW the plan. The advantage and peace of mind comes from accepting and believing in the plan. Our role is to watch it unfold and watch for the guideposts.

"We know that all things work together for the good of those who love God – those whom he has called according to his plan."
Romans 8:28 (God's Word)

Pastor Nathan Thompson gave a good description of how <u>The Purpose Driven Life</u> relates to all of us. This spoke particularly to me as I searched to understand the plan God had for me in relation to my cancer diagnosis. "He (Warren) simply believes that God in his sovereign wisdom knows our path and what ways we will choose. I heard someone say onetime that with God there is no "plan B." God allows us to make choices and decisions everyday about our lives, and in each choice, through his infinite wisdom, he knows how these choices will play out and affect our lives. That is why he wants us to follow him by faith, and to learn to know his purpose and will for us. For then in the choices we make we will find God's love, and joy, and fulfillment in many abundant ways." N. Thompson

"And when you draw close to God, God will draw close to you."
James 4:8a TLB

We want to know all and know the plan. Because if we knew the outcome (live or die) then we could feel in control again. If only we could make it our plan as we have managed and worked with our own plans before. Gods plan will unfold as God intended, whether we agree or not. Accepting guidance along the way will make the plan easier to "live" with.

"We should make plans – counting on God to direct us."
Proverbs 16:9 TLB

From the beginning, I believed that God's plan for me would be that I would survive this round of cancer. I was asked, "How did you know?" I didn't, I believed it and that grounded me. Outwardly others read this as a positive attitude or outlook. My spirit used this positive energy to move me forward. Believing God's plan, I could concentrate my energy on what was important and be far less distracted by minor issues.

God's plan for each of us is based on the multitude of promises he has made throughout the Bible, His word. These promises are between you and God. "Resist the temptation to try to figure out what it means for others. The Lord said it's none of your business. He wants your total surrender, your total trust, and that includes surrendering the need to know." Nelson pg. 68

We need a clear purpose to get up and get going every day. That purpose can be as basic as getting through the day in spite of feeling like a limp noodle, "one more day" chalked-off to recovery. God has greater purposes for each of us than merely making it through the day, unless the priority is to focus on healing. Then we need to work on the main purpose – healing is a cause and a prerequisite for all other intended purposes in life.

Believing that God's plan for me would be that I would recover was a motivator during cancer treatment and it still is today. Once I resigned myself that all this was not about me and I was not in control, I was able to become more receptive to seeking out guidance so I could stay on a path that would bring me to recovery. God has provided for medical technology and advancements. God has given physicians the intellect, skills and talents to bring this technology to us. To treat my cancer with anything less than the best and latest technology did not fit into my plan. I felt guided to my physicians and moved in many ways along a path that only spiritual help can explain.

"For I know the plans that I have for you, says the Lord. They are plans for good and not disaster, to give you a future with hope. " Jeremiah 29:11 TLB

God's plan is on its own time line. I felt like I hit a bonanza with the timing of my cancer. My first cancer surgery was scheduled on my birthday. That had benefits in that all the medical staff were extra nice to me. I'll never see that many birthday cards again until my 100th birthday. Chemotherapy treatments started in December and my hair fell out on Christmas Eve. December traditionally begins the flu season and with a past history of taking common colds to the flu stage and on to pneumonia, my doctor advised me to go into protective isolation and stay at home away from crowds. Chemo and radiation, both by default, drive a person's immunity to low levels and turn little sniffles into a huge threat. My spirit was a bit bummed to not be able to sing "Silent Night" at church on Christmas Eve as I was accustomed to doing. A group of cheerleaders from my church showed up at my door to sing Christmas carols right before Christmas and you bet I sang "Silent Night" with them. My spirit really appreciated that support. New Year's Eve morning brought another chemo treatment.

Protective isolation during the winter months in Minnesota feels a lot like house arrest. It gave a whole new meaning to 'cabin fever'. Every sunny afternoon, the Love Dog and I sprawled out on a recliner in front of the window and watched the snow sparkle. We are fortunate to have our home partially in the woods. We have beautiful landscape to contemplate and I soaked up the sun in peace and tranquility. My treatments were completed at the end of February 2004 and it was leap year. So that became my target celebration day, including a party for my cheerleaders on Leap Year Eve. I was then officially returning to the world with isolation over. "Celebrate everything" is my motto. Clever friends gave me 'leap back to life' gifts of frogs and other novelties to keep my spirit high. Snow in March became spring snow, as winter confinement was over and a new life of spring and recovery became a huge motivator.

There are increasing amounts of interest in research into understanding the restorative effects of religion and faith in healing. "Faith in God not only is epidemiologically significant but may be therapeutically significant as well. The role of faith and spirituality as a means of coping with existing physical or mental illness, and potentially hastening a cure, is an exciting frontier that physician-researchers are beginning to explore." Levin pg. 219.

SPIRIT

Now that we have entered a new world and have become 'the patient', the choices of treatment options are put in front of us. To do nothing to attempt to curtail the disease is always an option and a choice. Other choices will be more aggressive and potential side effects will be explained. I encourage you to ask questions until you have the confidence to understand every option. Personally, I was one who dreaded surprises and felt much better knowing exactly what was coming and what to expect. Others roll with the punches better than I do. I found there is far more stress packed into the unknown which is just another way of saying 'Knowledge is Power'. While waiting to hear the report of lab results, I referred to this as *The Unknown Zone*. When friends asked how I was doing during these high anxiety times of waiting for results, I had to reply that I was in the Zone again. Good supporters always checked back.

We all have expectations of health care which are both good and bad. Who hasn't heard a horror story of what went wrong somewhere to somebody? Prior to a major illness, we had been accustomed to the 'fix and go' plan in terms of health care.

As a child, I got strep throat at least once every winter. My mom called the same pediatrician every time and then would pick up the prescription. Within 24 hours of choking down that nasty tasting pink goop, the soreness would ease and I could move up from Popsicles to ice cream and the next day it was back to hot dogs. We will get to guided imagery later, but, I no longer can type about the pink goop without the taste getting in my mouth – yuk! Imagery is a wonderful technique. The pattern or expectation of 'fix and go' was then learned – get sick, get medicine, get better.

I was dutifully cleaning my girls' goldfish bowl one day when I scrubbed a thin spot on the glass and my thumb went right through. (As an aside, why is this a mom's job?) Anyway, lots of blood, nice gash and obvious need for a few stitches and to clean the algae out of my thumb tissue. So, into the doctor, get the cleaning, a few stitches, tetanus shot and back home. A week later, I was able to clean out the new plastic fish bowl with the same hand. It still entertains me to this day that two people actually asked me if the fish died when the bowl broke. I was under the assumption fish would not like soap in their water, so had given them temporary confinement in a cereal bowl.

It is not a surprise that once confronted with a major illness like cancer, ALS or a chronic condition such as diabetes or MS, our mindset is not initially thinking beyond our past experience. We expect we can visit the doctor and get the cure, the fix, the stitches and BINGO – back to life as it was. There is an adjustment to the new reality that has to happen. It is definitely not an upbeat feeling but necessary, just the same, to be able to move forward to the goal of successful treatment.

It is at this point where trust in your physician becomes critical. We have to trust that the best options have been put in front of us. We need to believe in the unseen and know that reason alone will not get us on the right path to a cure. A miracle cure may be developed and become a regular protocol for treatment in just 2 years. But, it's not available to you today; it is not part of your decision and not part of today's possibilities. We have to work with what we have. There is a point where you know you have gathered all the information possible. Comfort to move ahead with a course of treatment may well take a leap of faith. It's time to cozy up to your Spirit. Jesus promised us a Counselor to be with us forever – the Holy Spirit:

"Spirit of truth. The world cannot accept him, because it neither sees nor knows him, for he lives with you and will be in you."
John 14:17 NIV

In describing Spiritual Warriors, "It is the warrior's soul that gives direction to his mind and strength to his body." (Weber pg. 57)

"...We know that suffering creates endurance, endurance creates character, and character creates confidence. We're not ashamed to have this confidence, because God's love has been poured into our hearts by the Holy Spirit, who has been given to us." Romans 5:3-5 (God's Word)

If you believe God has a plan for you, you have to gain the feeling that you are in sync with the plan. It's a need to feel the guidance and to know it is right. This is what leads to peace of mind and the belief that your decisions were right. I had to listen intently and look closely for God's signs. We live in an age of multi media and movies with special effects. We've been somewhat conditioned by this extreme noise to fail to hear the soft whisper. Do we look for fireworks in the sky and miss the small candle for light? It would be easier to just follow along behind a booming command, but who said it would be easy?

"...but the mind controlled by the Spirit is life and peace."
Romans 8:6b NIV

In prayer, meditation, and all relaxation techniques, the stress of the daily world, the noises and all the other interruptions to mentally focus need to be put aside. Only then can you hear the soft whisper of the spirit within you. Through imagery I learned to use mind visuals to help me see my spirit. I could then read the body language of my spirit with the universal 'come to me' motions of open arms and hands beckoning to me. Being a visual person and daughter of an artist, this was my easiest level for connection to my spirit. Others have felt a nudge, heard the soft whisper and envisioned their spirit in a number of ways. Experiencing the presence of your spirit is much more important than how.

"God didn't give us a cowardly spirit but a spirit of power, love, and good judgment."
2 Timothy 1:7 (God's Word)

A Cherokee Proverb: One evening an old Cherokee told his grandson about a battle that goes on inside people. He said, "My son, the battle is between two wolves. One is Evil. It is anger, envy, sorrow, regret, greed, arrogance, self-pity, guilt, resentment, infe-riority, lies, false pride, superiority and ego. The other is Good. It is joy, peace, love, hope, serenity, humility, kindness, benevolence, empathy, generosity, truth, compassion and faith." The grandson thought about it for a minute and then asked his grandfather, "Which wolf wins?" The old Cherokee simply replied, "The one you feed." It's time to start nurturing your spirit.

"…He (God) will strengthen you with power through his Spirit in your inner being." Ephesians 3:16b NIV

"The emerging medical model postulates that body, mind and something beyond mind – call it 'spirit' – work together to promote health, prevent illness and produce healing." Levin pg. 207. With the big decisions to make in front of you, take a 'time out' and listen closely to your spirit. God is ready and waiting to speak to you through your spirit and when you embrace it, the marvelous peace of mind will both comfort you and lift you up.

"When I called, you answered me. You made me bold by strengthening my soul."
Psalm 138:3 (God's Word)

ON THE PATH

W hether you have decided against having treatment for the disease, or embarking on a treatment plan, the path ahead will be a long one. I sure missed the days of the quick health fixes. An extended time frame is a daunting proposition. My physician told me many times that all was temporary. Any side effects and even hair loss is only temporary. My spirit picked up on the word 'temporary' and used it often to motivate me.

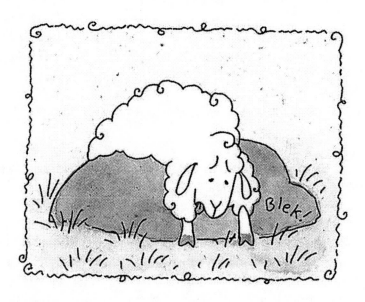

Cancer treatments, including chemotherapy and radiation, require time to work as designed. The intensity of the chemo drugs and the radiation process target, and ideally destroy, the cancer cells. The fallout, of course, is the damage done to surrounding cells and tissue. I referred to the good ones as perfectly innocent cells just minding their own business. The healthy cells take a few hits, but they will come back with nurturing and get on with life – that's what they do best. We need to be a patient and think 'temporary'.

"Trust the Lord with all your heart, and do not rely on your own understanding. In all your ways acknowledge him, and he will make your paths smooth." Proverbs 3:5-6(God's Word)

First, we trust our medical team to provide us the best options and accept that our level of understanding exactly how treatments will work will never compare to the trained professionals. Keep your focus on the highest priority of completing treatment or reaching the end goal. And most importantly, feel the relief that God's plan for you is in action and trust in the Lord and let his spirit guide you to the smooth path. If still feeling a bit shaky about your decision or the path you have chosen, scripture tells us to:

"Wait with hope for the Lord, Be strong, and let your heart be courageous. Yes, wait with hope for the Lord." Psalm 27:14 (God's Word)

"Be strong and take heart, all you who hope in the Lord.." Psalm 31:24 NIV

Be good to yourself. If entering an aggressive treatment, remember those innocent healthy cells and give them a break. All treatments drain your energy, so ease up on the stress of everyday life as treatment will be stress enough. Prepare to take a sabbatical from life as you know it. Some treatments allow for maintaining a normal work schedule and others will require mega amounts of time to heal. It's best to prepare to cutback by assuring the door is open to taper even further if needed. Do your best to make no commitments on any large scale until treatment is completed. Since we are used to managing our own business, it is stressful when we cannot live up to our commitments. Even low-key commitments created excess anxiety for me as I feared I would not have the energy to fulfill what I had promised to do. Eventually, I figured out that just about everything can be postponed, or at least delegated, and I saved plans for when I had recovered. It felt good to get rid of the clutter and feel unobstructed momentum on the path to recovery. Who knew there would be so many others to carry life's baggage for me?!

In his book, Timeless Healing, Dr. Benson gives some wonderful insights into healing and life transformation. With 25 years of experience as a physician and researcher, he was one of the first to write about the mind/body/spirit connection from a physician's viewpoint. Dr. Benson gives numerous examples of how positive energy affects health. He notes particularly that belief in a higher power will make a contribution to physical health. What struck me most about his beliefs is that he describes how we are 'wired for God'. Prayer and meditation nourish us. Dr. Benson suggests that combining age-old faith, the wisdom of modern medicine and the aid of a caring physician will heal over 60% of medical problems. He has done a great deal to bring the faith community and the scientific world closer together.

It was easy to get testimonies from the doctors at my clinic. They all know of patients who had cancer with terrible prognosis who surprised everyone when they beat the cancer. They told me that medically, there is absolutely no reason some people should still be alive and yet they come in for check-ups and convince us over and over again that faith is real and makes a huge difference in outcomes.

We all know of people with positive attitudes and goals who are cancer survivors. True to Dr. Benson's writing, the person in treatment with the positive attitude also gives off positive energy to those around them. It is the difference between expressing how bad you feel that your friend needs another surgery, to responding with "Glad to hear the expected result of the surgery will help stop the disease. You are making progress. Let's celebrate!" The positive energy sent out elicits positive vibes in response. Whenever I laughed, I knew

I was giving others permission to laugh with me and lighten the mood. For example, some women look spectacular bald, not me. Rather than having supporters express how they felt sorry for me when I needed to wear a wig, why not laugh at the reality and toast to it being temporary.

Dr. Benson does a wonderful job of explaining how our expectations of treatment will influence us. Chemotherapy drugs have long lists of potential side effects. Will being too familiar with possible side effects cause us to get the side effects? Being informed is important as some side effects require medical attention and need to be managed properly. So many factors come into play including each person's uniqueness. Trust your physician and medical team to guide you in managing the medical issues as they arise.

"(The Lord says,) I will instruct you. I will teach you the way that you should go. I will advise you as my eyes watch over you." Psalm 32:8 (God's Word)

Once on the treatment path, all of us basic managers, and especially those like me who lean towards the 'control-freak' side, realize we just can't do all this alone. We must let the Lord take charge. I know the Lord kept close company with my spirit and was a solid companion at all times including times when I was rolled into an operating room. The other people in the operating room were strangers to me but my spirit was there and acted almost as a buffer to be my wide-awake companion – I went quickly to land of the fog. To feel that healthy spirit watching over your sick body relieves a lot of stress. This stress relief is even measurable with lower blood pressure and lower heart rate. Those masked people in the operating rooms love that!

"Wait calmly for God alone, my soul, because my hope comes from him." Psalm 62:5 (God's Word)

"Because God wanted to make the unchanging nature of his purpose very clear to the heirs of what was promised, he confirmed it with an oath. God did this so that, by two

unchangeable things in which it is impossible for God to lie, we who have fled to seize the hope offered to us may be greatly encouraged. We have the hope as an anchor for the soul, firm and secure." Hebrews 6:17 – 19 NIV

About this verse, Stu Weber's comment was: "Two unchangeable things: a promise and an oath – both based on the integrity and character of God Himself, Wow –that's strong encouragement! Encouragement to do what? To seize the hope! Get hold of it! It's incredible! It's true. It's certain. It's guaranteed. It's eternal. Seize it and hang on." Pg. 177. Try to recognize what gets you down or eats away at your positive energy and outlook. Then run the other way.

When undergoing treatment, we have to think in terms of a prognosis. A prognosis is loaded with uncertainty and a long-time commitment in the 'unknown zone'. I found it too easy to build up a mountain of negative energy and fresh stress dwelling on the prognosis. It was far better to embrace what I believed to be certain and bask in the glow of positive energy.

"We live by faith, not by sight." 2 Corinthians 5:7 NIV

The initial fears that come packaged with a serious health diagnosis can be replaced with courage when put into perspective. The more we pray, focus and meditate on looking for the path God wants us to follow, the clearer the right way becomes. The fog lifts. Seeing the path clearly is the best motivator to keep going, to follow without question and know it's the right way to go. You're not out there alone – the Holy Spirit is beside you and dwelling within you. Hope stays renewed and the positive energy you feel keeps the strength and courage coming. God has a plan for each of us that is constant and unchanging from day to day. We each also have a purpose in life. While we cannot see what lies ahead, we are left to trust that God will direct our steps along the way.

"...Wait for the Lord, and he will come and save you! Be brave, stouthearted and courageous. Yes, wait and he will help you." Psalm 27:14 TLB

The Bible makes many references to God's word being a light to guide his people. Stress, worry, anxiety, fear and negative energy all fit into biblical use of 'darkness' of life. Move to the light every opportunity you have and shine in it.

"O Lord, you light my lamp. My God turns my darkness into light." Psalm 18:28 (God's Word)

"Your word is a lamp to my feet and a light for my path." Psalm 119:105 NIV

The treatment path appears long and endless, especially in the beginning. By looking forward, the path will look a little shorter every day – and it is! When little else seems positive, embrace your progress and celebrate everything you can. By letting my spirit be in charge of directing my steps, I was able to stay positive and know it was the right way to go.

"If the Lord delights in a man's way, he makes his steps firm; though he stumble, he will not fall, ..." Psalm 37:23 NIV

PERSONALLY SUPPORTING YOUR SPIRIT & BODY

"Don't be afraid, because I am with you. Don't be intimidated; I am your God. I will strengthen you. I will help you. I will support you with my victorious right hand." Isaiah 41:10 (God's Word)

For those of us who consider ourselves independent, self-sufficient and tough, a major health crisis may well be the wake-up call we need. A lengthy treatment plan is even longer for those who go it alone. Even in those lonely times when I was home and physically miserable, my healthy spirit kept me company. I knew my spirit was being supported at all times as it is God's assurance that even when our body is not strong, our spirit is. Spiritual strength is a gift of grace and readily available.

Ideally, each person has a support network in place with faith, family and friends. Realizing the importance of support is critical, as facing cancer alone is stressful and a much harder path to travel. I was with my Bible study group of friends when I needed to leave early for a first biopsy appointment. Knowing my risk factors were definitely high, I certainly was not looking forward to this procedure, but thought I was tough enough to go on my own. My friend, Beth, offered at least three times to go along that day and be my buddy. I was bred to be stoic and self-sufficient, but deep inside I feared I might need her help more in the future. That was an unfounded fear

I learned later. I turned Beth down and marched off by myself. A procedure that should have taken 30 minutes lasted much longer as all had not gone smoothly. By the time I came out into the hospital lobby wearing my new ace bandage bra (under my shirt I looked like a uni-boob with mega cleavage, although no one noticed), I was fully convinced that a breast cancer diagnosis was just a lab test away. The radiologist who had done the procedure had been honest and referred to the biopsy as 'highly suspicious'. There I was, by myself, strung high on anxiety and regretting that I'd been so foolish to blow off Beth's genuine offer of friendship and support.

My mother used to take my brother and me for an ice cream cone as a payoff for being good when we got vaccinations or had other doctor visits. It was special treat when only my brother had gotten a shot. I had been good during the biopsy so I bought myself an updated version – a big smoothie from the hospital snack bar. There I sat like a limp noodle in the lobby, hoping the smoothie would work its magic and I would mellow enough to get in my car and go home. Desperately I wished Beth were there – anything to not be alone at that point.

"Two can accomplish more than twice as much as one…If one falls when he is alone, he's in trouble." Ecclesiastes 4:9-10 TLB

That biopsy appointment was my wake up call and maybe the lesson I needed to learn. Support from family and friends are critical. Reach out and ask for help – it's the only way to cope and survive the hard times. I confessed to Beth that I'd been a fool to turn down her offer of support. Dear friend that she is, Beth only replied, "I like smoothies." And for me, lesson learned!

"A person's anxiety will weigh him down, but an encouraging word makes him joyful." Proverbs 12:25 (God's Word)

Support and acts of Christian love are pure ENCOURAGEMENT – the best of gifts. Having learned my lesson when I did not accept Beth's support when offered, I knew I would have to keep my supporters informed of my progress. With each lab test, surgery and treatment, those who are offering support both want and really need to know what is happening. It is absolutely exhausting to get on the phone and make many calls each time. Friends also chose to not call me as they knew I needed to rest and they respected that. So, I got in the habit of sending an e-mail update. A typical one read, "I got run over by that big truck (chemo treatment session) yesterday, but have managed to crawl to the curb already. Thanks for your prayers." This short note was then forwarded to many others. Later in the day, and for the next few days, most of them responded with further words of encouragement. I was always connected.

"When I kept things to myself, I felt weak deep inside me." Psalm 32:3 (God's Word)

I referred to my supporters as my cheerleaders. From 'hang in there' statements to countdowns, they remained very creative and did what they could to keep my spirit happy as well as healthy. Humor seemed a bit limited during chemotherapy, so keeping the spirit happy was a challenge. Countdowns like 'one quarter done,' 'half done,' 'three quarters done' gave opportunity for cheers. We focused only on the positive, so my glass was half-full, rather than half empty. Groups of friends and whole families came together to support my spirit. They reaffirmed their commitment to each other and to me. Each one was nearer and dearer than I ever could have imagined before my cancer experience. I have been blessed with a classic 'cup runneth over' life.

SUPPORTING OUR OWN SPIRITS

POWER OF PRAYER
"The Lord is near to all who call on him..." Psalm 145:18a NIV

A health crisis is stress enough. There is absolutely nothing to be gained from trying to tough it out on your own. Through prayer God's comfort reaches you and restores your inner positive energy. God cares about you and waits with open arms to accept all your worries. God knows our every worry and concern, so prayer needs no explanation. We want to be healed. For the healing to begin, we need to reach out and ask God for His help. The Lord is always near and readily available, but each person needs to take the action to request help in healing.

"Let him (God) have all your worries and cares, for he is always thinking about you and watching everything that concerns you."
1 Peter 5:7 TLB

The Bible assures us that we are free from fighting. Fighting sounds too much like a battle to me. Our job is to pray and wait patiently. In Exodus 14:14, it is straightforward.

"Remain calm; the Lord will fight for you."

All we need to do is trust and the Lord will fight for us. Trust the Lord to be in control as he knows His plan for each of us. To believe this relieves the stress of the unknown and the calm peace of mind soothes body and spirit.

"The prayer offered in faith will make the sick person well: The Lord will raise him up...."
James 5:15 NIV

"At the same time the Spirit also helps us in our weakness, because we don't know how to pray for what we need. But the Spirit intercedes along with our groans that cannot be expressed in words. The one who searches our hearts knows what the Spirit has in mind. The Spirit intercedes for God's people the way God wants him to." Romans 8:26-27 (God's Word)

Feeling my own spirit connected and in touch with the Holy Spirit was powerful. It's a gift of grace to have the Holy Spirit present mentoring our own spirits. Accepting by faith that God is the only one in control, the Holy Spirit helps to manage, not control our thoughts and fears. At the height of my health crisis, I knew I had over 500 Christians praying for me in at least seven states. That was awesome! Words cannot describe the feeling.

I was specific in asking for prayers to get me safely through surgery. In the minutes until anesthesia takes over, I let my mind think about specific people praying for me at that moment. I thought I would see faces. Rather than faces I saw almost a glow and an aura surround me like a mist of protection. I was confident I was safe and it was secure protection. In addition, I used imagery to see my own spirit standing next to me with the Holy Spirit looking over my spirit's shoulder. I would be unconscious, but I had two personal attendants on guard providing for my protection. All the prayers from others would hold them there and I was not alone in the operating room.

Again, I have to appreciate the high-speed benefits of e-mail. It was primarily through e-mail that I could let my prayer supporters all over the country know of my specific requests and when I needed their prayers. Even our prayer chain at our church uses e-mail. My good friend, Marie James, would call her dad when she e-mailed or phoned me. Before surgeries, her parents would call me and pray with me over the phone. Her father was the pastor who confirmed me in the Lutheran faith, officiated at my wedding and baptized my two daughters. It was a gift of security and meant so much.

"...I (Lord) have heard your prayer and seen your tears; I will heal you..." 2 Kings 20:5b NIV

If you have a church home, call and connect yourself with their prayer ministry program. If you are not connected at present or would like to expand your horizons on the power of prayer, look on the website www.prayerventures.org for wonderful information for "Reaching, refreshing, healing and empowering through Christ" with prayer. Books, CDs and schedules of seminars are also available on the website. In her book, The Healing Moment, Betsy Lee offers an "invitation to enter fully into God's presence – to take time to discover the gift of healing and acceptance that God longs to give us."

While on the topic of prayer, I kept all my prayers directed to God, the Holy Spirit and/or Christ. I have heard others relate how they gave credit to their guardian angels. Stu Weber offers these guidelines and cautions.

"1. Never let your imagination shape your understanding of angels.

Broadly speaking, most of what you will see, hear, and read concerning angels in contemporary literature is the product of active human imagination – not solid biblical reality. If you want the straight scoop on these powerful allies of God's people, go directly to the Bible, not coffee table books, magazines, or tabloids.

2. Never let your heart pursue angels in place of God in your life.

This is a constant temptation for people because of our natural fascination with the unseen world around us. Angels are real. They are also created beings. They are not God. The first of the Ten Commandments makes it clear that you must have "no other gods" before Him! Know God, not angels. Study your Lord, not His messengers. And that leads to the ultimate caution.

3. Never let your soul worship angels.

Never give them glory, honor, or worship. They are mere creatures. The evil one, himself an angel (albeit fallen), would love to divert you from the Living One." Pg. 113.

NUTRITION

A nutritionist for many years, I was surprised during my experience with cancer that very limited nutritional advice was offered. I am a practical person and will not engage you in a long nutrition discussion in this book. Select carefully what and whom you chose to believe. Many have made millions promoting the nutritional benefits of various foods, eating protocols like diets, supplements and herbs, anti-cancer regimens, and so on. Know you can trust the source, question even more if a product or book is being sold, ask your physician for clarification and be sure your physician is aware of any supplement you are taking outside of what he has prescribed.

Be sensible and use common sense to meet your nutritional needs. The goal of chemotherapy drugs and radiation is to destroy the cancer cells. With these treatments, normal healthy cells are also harmed. Our bodies frantically work to repair and replace these good cells. When the repair job is done, we are healthy again. This takes energy and basic, good nutrition.

When we do not feel well and/or are nauseated, it is unrealistic to think every meal will be perfectly balanced. Taking a daily multivitamin is without question. We require protein to build new cells. On days when too nauseated to eat solids, I lived on Ensure drinks and worked my way up to dairy products to get the most protein possible. People cautioned me that I wouldn't like the taste of meat, but I found that on good days, even red meat was acceptable. We are individuals and own our own tastes. I very deliberately pushed protein in all forms so I could feel proactive in helping myself heal. Protein rich foods also provide iron which will slow the anemia side effects.

Like many, I felt full on very small portions and always felt better if I ate a good protein snack like a cheese stick, hard-boiled egg or yogurt between meals. Scrambled eggs or French toast was easy to prepare and rich in protein. Friends brought me delicious homemade soups.

Juices, while acidic, were fine as long as I was eating some other foods at the time. Besides the emphasis on protein, Vitamin C from juices or fruits helps with the healing and provides a defense against infection. Huge doses of Vitamin C or other vitamins or minerals may be asking for trouble by triggering other side effects.

Healthy diets include whole grains as a main source of carbohydrates. Raw vegetables and many raw fruits, while marvelous for those dieting as they help you to feel full, do take more metabolic energy to break down in digestion. For a stomach already stressed and possibly aggravated by treatments, stick with cooked vegetables and canned fruits for easier digestion. I conserved metabolic energy wherever I could without neglecting nutritional basics.

Nutrition is a science based on scientific research. It is a complimentary care, not a cure. While in treatment for cancer, the goal is to maintain your current weight. To intentionally work on weight loss, forces your body to try to heal using waste products. When we lose weight, the excess fat that is being burned up for energy leaves waste products in the blood. This is manageable by a healthy body, but a body tolerating treatment and trying to repair itself does much better without waste in the way. A body trying to heal is craving proteins and all the essential building blocks. An empty stomach can feel more irritated. It is often recommended to try to eat small meals or healthy snacks often versus a large meal. To snack more often can lead to some weight gain and most physicians will accept a little weight gain over loss during treatment. If you fear weight gain, consider a low fat cheese stick for a snack instead of a dish of ice cream, a peanut butter cracker rather than a candy bar, etc.

Expect a heightened sense of smell and use for the benefit of a 'Happy Tummy' (term is courtesy of my brother). My husband was good enough to curb his love of Cajun cooking. Memorie, my neighbor, brought me loaves of homemade wheat bread still warm – heaven!

NUTRITIONAL SUPPLEMENTS

Nutrition is a science. It is neither an opinion nor a testimonial. Before taking ANY supplement, be informed and get your physician's approval. It is not fair to a physician to withhold the information on your supplement intake. Statistically, it is reported that one third of all cancer patients take supplements regularly unbeknownst to their physician. Personally, I think that is a low estimate.

Unfortunately, no list of herbs with known harmful effects or anti-cancer benefits exists as it changes daily. The following are questions you should always ask before taking any supplement:

1. Will the supplement interfere with any of my prescribed medications? This is the primary reason to clear supplements with your physician.
2. Are testimonials from well meaning people the reason I want to try this supplement OR is there a reliable scientific basis?
3. Is it worth the money?
4. Are you getting the recommended amounts of nutrients in your diet including your basic multivitamin? Is there really a need to supplement or provide excess amounts? Supplement quantities are not regulated, making it easy to over dose.

The bottom line is to be both informed as to the value of any supplement and get your physician's approval. See the Internet Recourses Guide under "Supplements." Medical professionals subscribe to the Natural Medicine Database at www.naturaldatabase.com listing most herbs and supplements, mechanism of action, safety, side effects and interactions. All the latest data is listed. Nothing is being sold at the site.

REST AND SLEEP

"I fall asleep in peace the moment I lie down because you alone, O Lord, enable me to live securely." Psalm 4:8 (God's Word)

Sleep is so basic to life and sometimes so hard to get.

The National Sleep Foundation website, www.sleepfoundation. org, reports results from their annual sleep surveys of Americans. In 2005, only 26% of Americans reported getting 8 hours of sleep on weekdays, down from 38% in 2001. In the 1950s, over 95% would get 8 hours of sleep on weekdays. This data raises issues on what happens to our general health if we are not adequately giving the body time to rest and repair itself. After a short night when maybe you were up with a sick child and only got 2 hours of sleep, how was your mental function the next day? There is concern and a great deal of data coming out on the effects of lack of sleep and driving ability. Vehicle accidents are increasingly caused by sleepy drivers who have the slower reflexes or worse, actually fall asleep behind the wheel.

The bottom line is that we all need to do what it takes to get a full eight hours of sleep. It actually stresses the body to deprive it of necessary rest and sleep. At my house, we referred to it as putting the baby (me) to bed by 8 p.m. Friends knew not to call me after 8. Instead, they would send me an e-mail, knowing I could read it and respond when I wanted a conversation and was awake. My husband could still watch television or be on the phone behind a door and he made the effort to keep the house quiet for me. To protect my sleep time, I also needed to make barriers for night noises while being hospitalized. I put a relaxation CD on continuous play, but, being a light sleeper, I ended up listening for the end of one piece and anticipating the next. A nurse, who had just ordered a white noise sound machine for herself, recommended I check the www. marpac.com website. It was an excellent suggestion. I use the sound machine only occasionally now, but it is still useful when traveling to miss hearing the hotel hallway doors close.

"Come to me, all who are tired from carrying heavy loads, and I will give you rest." Matthew 11:28 (God's Word)

Evening rituals to prepare your body for rest and sleep are important. Some have hot tea, take a long, leisurely bath, read to get drowsy, drink warm milk, stay in a darkened room with minimal light to gain from the melatonin effect, take calcium supplements at bedtime to help regulate sleep patterns, or eat a turkey snack that provides tryptophan (amino acid - chemical that makes us drowsy on Thanksgiving Day). The other side is to avoid eating late in the day, alcohol, caffeine, heavy exercise, loud music or anything that normally keeps you awake. Early on give in to this need for sleep and rest as it's vital in helping you heal, cope and recover. Sleep deprivation is an extremely difficult side effect to manage. I know this intimately – avoid it at all costs.

We all wish we could sleep as peacefully as a baby. With a full, happy tummy, babies sleep without worry or care. Think of the children's prayers that so simply state we are free to sleep because God will be watching over and caring for us. End your evening prayers with reaffirming to yourself that God will watch over you and take over your worries and fears so you can sleep and feel rested. Mary brought me little treats weekly. She brought me the following saying written in fancy calligraphy: "Give your troubles to God. He's up all night anyway." It's framed and next to my bed when I need the reminder.

JOURNALING
Keeping a journal has become very popular as a way to help deal with sorrows, stress, illness and many other of life's problems. A cancer diagnosis, barrage of treatment choices, upside down family plans, new needs with less independence, work and family commitments and more thrown into a heap of disorganized brain clutter left me reeling.

"Expressive writing" is another common term for journaling which better describes our attempt to put our emotions into words. Once in words and thought through piece by piece, the clutter is replaced with more understanding and we begin to put behind us the unsettling thoughts. Being able to express your feelings in writing is definitely a release valve and will help keep everything in perspective. Serious reflection on what is happening to you is tremendously beneficial in embracing the big picture. You also see more clearly what you have accomplished and what is behind you. You gain the sense of momentum of moving forward and progressing to the end of treatment. Progress in and of itself is a motivator and good, positive energy.

While receiving treatment, I had the opportunity to attend a short class on journaling, one I passed up. Ah, to live and learn. I can only imagine how much easier writing this book would have been if I had done a journal.

BLOGGING

P. Bergman, MD founded a website, www.RedToeNail.org to be available to people whose lives have been touched by cancer as a patient or as a caregiver or friend. "Your blog is your story – the good, the bad and the ugly. But it is an important story for your family, friends and loved ones." Bergman. This can be a supportive online environment where you share your experiences in blog versus journal format. For some it has been a place to learn from others and find support for their challenges.

VISUALIZATION

Dr. Phil (McGraw) made the idea of visualization known with his philosophy on successful weight loss. For weight loss, he suggested holding an image of yourself in your mind's eye of how you will realistically look IF you lose weight. That is with the smaller, trimmer waistline, smaller size clothes, the thinner legs, etc. This is only part of his plan. It has merit in that if you are trying to lose weight and visualize the preferred body shape, you may well be able to stop yourself from those food indiscretions that will keep you from attaining the new shape.

You need no special training to use this same technique while being treated for a disease. I was bald with dark circles under my eyes and my skin was the color of lutefisk. (A male friend provided me this skin color description after, thankfully, my normal skin color returned and meant it as a compliment.) The all too real, perfect reflection in the mirror did nothing to brighten my day. I am quite sure my healthy spirit kept me away from mirrors where an unhealthy body would stare back. It was far more therapeutic for me to think about my goal of my hair growing back, no dark circles and a healthy, glowing suntan. In your mind you can have a wonderful suntan without skin cancer or wrinkle threat. Personally, I became touchy about being in a photograph. This was hardly a challenge when firmly planted at home on protective isolation. There's only one photo of me with my wig on and that is one too many. Looking at pre-sick photo albums did lift me up and nurtured my visualizing of how I would look again when my temporary status of treatment ended. Let the positive energy flow.

IMAGERY

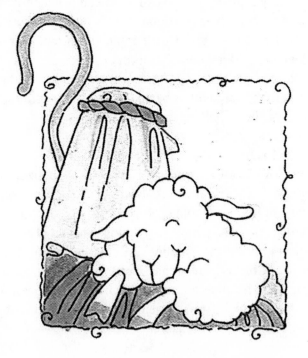

Similar to visualization, using imagery is a wonderful technique to calm stress. The drawing on page 58 was on a greeting card. I was almost mesmerized by its simple lines depicting such a huge message.

He tends his flock like a shepherd: He gathers the lambs in his arms and carries them close to his heart;" Isaiah 40:11a NIV

I was the little lamb in need of a good shepherd to carry me. I tucked the card into my hospital bag and headed off for another surgery. Jodie was my pre-surgery companion for the trip and I shared the card with her so she would know my imagery plan for the day. When ready to roll down the hall to the surgery suite, the nursing staff directed Jodie to the waiting area. She lingered in the doorway so I would see her caressing the weak, frightened lamb she pretended to hold. Imagery works, and having a caring friend make it a real visual is incredible.

We are all God's children. There are many images in paintings and drawings where Jesus is with children. When fears mount, flip through some of those remembered pictures in your mind. See yourself as one of the children in the comfort of Jesus. Imagery is easy and effective.

PERKS OF PETS

Dr. Marty Becker of Ohio is a veterinarian who fully recognizes the healing power of pets and wrote a delightful book filled with heart touching stories. "Part of the healing power of pets is their capacity to make the atmosphere safe for emotions, the spiritual side of healing. Whatever you're feeling, you can express it around your pet. Let it out, let it go and not be judged for it. In that way, we don't have to censor ourselves around our beloved four-legged friends, nor do we censor our feelings for them when they get sick. …..a capacity to have the emotional impact of disease, something that all too frequently is shoved under the rug in the treatment of cancer in humans. When you know your caregiver is afraid and is being touched by that fear, it hurts both." Pg. 80.

My Love Dog was only 11 weeks old when she made a clumsy fall off our rain coated slippery deck into a mud puddle below. A back leg snapped ending up in a cast. To console our whimpering, sad-eyed little puppy, my daughters and I (my husband still denies it) would rock her to sleep in our laps. Six years and 64 pounds later, we have no reason to wonder how she ended up to be a lap dog. She's well trained in the art of comfort sharing.

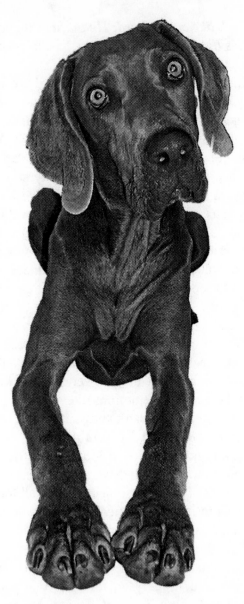

Listening without judgment makes pets ideal companions for anyone with a serious or chronic illness. By talking about the illness/trauma that upset our life, it helps us deal with the stress of the whole situation. Pets love to hear the story as often as you tell it. The family, friends and caregivers who already know the story get a break. They are saved from having to mention they have heard it before or roll their eyes up in their heads. Pets understand you need to repeat it and they will listen again and again.

Pets crave being touched and are happy to return soothing tactile comfort to the giver. Many of the chronic diseases and cancers are not contagious. Yet, human's deep-seated fears, some unconscious, make us reluctant to touch those who are ill. Those of us who undergo cancer treatment, with its side effect of depressed immunity protection, get into the reverse situation. I was on protective isolation and cautioned to avoid human touch for fear of picking up a virus. My supporters were totally respectful of this. Another reason to keep them informed. No one brought a cold or flu bug into my house. In lieu of real hugs, we did e-mail and air hugs – it helped fill the void.

During an illness, it gnaws on our psyche to feel dependence on others while missing dearly our usual, healthy independence. Having a pet offers some physical exercise and the opportunity to provide care and love for another while boosting our own positive energy and self-image. Some of the anger, stress or resentment is channeled in a positive way while caring for the pet. Offering some pet help is a good way to support someone, especially if they live alone and do not have the ability to take their pet out for a walk, to the groomer, etc. My Love Dog was relieved to have my husband play rough and offer physical exercise in the evenings after a long day of caring and listening to me. I feel obligated to confess her eyes did roll up in her head more than once.

Studies on pets have also shown the benefit of decreasing human pain by the mere act of petting. "By initiating and maintaining the relaxation response, pets can take people's focus off of their pain and elevate their moods. Secondly, through touch or physical contact, they can block the transmission of their pain from the periphery to the central nervous system, shutting the pain-processing centers down." Becker pg. 106.

To pet a dog's head with a gentle touch and fingertips seems to be universally enjoyed by all dogs. Their eyes get dreamy and they beam serenity. As a side note, when my pre-hair fuzz started to grow in after temporary baldness ended, it was very thick and ultra soft, like marvelous rich velvet. Those who saw it routinely begged to touch it. Why not, if it gives them a thrill, it was the least I could do after the support they'd given me. For a human, petting my head hair just did not feel the same as dogs must experience. If it hadn't all been in fun, it might have felt a bit freaky!

I am hopeful allergies or your current living arrangement does not forbid pets. If you are looking to be a new pet owner while receiving treatment, a mature pet would be a better choice than a puppy. Visiting pets at nursing homes provide lots of comfort therapy. If friends are coming to visit you, invite them to bring their pet along. Pets offer us a bond with all of nature. Dr. Becker summed it up best, "They (pets) take us outside of ourselves and reacquaint us with the world we live in. Our need for each other, which is part spiritual, part visceral, helps keep us happy and healthy." Pg. 254

HUMOR

Medical treatments in and of themselves offer few opportunities for genuine humor. It takes a little effort, but if you look, you'll find some. Jan drove me to some medical appointments and purposely saved up her bizarre milkman stories. She was able to entertain me for three hours while I was getting chemo. Want her phone number?

A guaranteed source of humor is being bald, unless you happen to be one of the women who look spectacular bald. Go with the belief that laughing helps hair to grow back faster. Christine Clifford's No Hair Day book is sure to bring a smile. Most of the women I know have at least one funny story concerning their wig. My daughter was two steps behind me when I walked into a store with her. The air lock between the inner and outer doors sucked my wig right off my head. Feeling the breeze, I spun around in horror only to see her burst out laughing. To this day, mention that store name and she starts to laugh. She claims she will never forget the look on my face or be able to enter those doors without the memory. To finish the story, I dove to the dirty floor and in my haste put the wig on backwards before standing up. By then we both had tears from laughing so hard. Who cares? We are not sure anyone else was an eyewitness – too bad, it was hilarious.

Humor helps keep you grounded. Sharing a chuckle with my physician is doubly therapeutic.

MUSIC

Most of us enjoy music in one form or another to brighten our day. We routinely have the car radio or CDs on to help us through the rush hour traffic. When home alone and doing mundane tasks, music is great company. Singing along makes the house cleaning go faster. In general, music provides for us a mental health break, takes the edge off the stress of the day, and of course, is enjoyable. It makes sense to incorporate music into your healing journey. Music can affect emotions, behavior and even physiology. It's known to settle restless thinking, lessen worry and promote relaxation.

There is an abundance of relaxation and wellness CDs available today, from gentle nature sounds of waves, birds singing, and rainfall to human compositions designed just for relaxation. This type of music is ideal for background music during meditation. Music by itself is excellent when you are too tired to read or engage in any activity.

Andrew Lloyd Weber's composition of "Music of the Night " from Phantom of the Opera illustrates beautifully the idea of surrendering to the music. It is with a surrender feeling that you can listen to music and hear so much more than you had before. Particularly with soft Christian music, you may hear words you did not before as we dig in deeper than flowing with the melody. The very act of surrendering during a health crisis comes up often. In more ways than one we let go of some of our need to control and allow someone else to guide us. I was all excited about the letting go concept and asked my Bible study group of 50 women to try to embrace the surrender feeling by listening with their eyes closed to Andre Bocelli and Celine Dion:

THE PRAYER

I pray you'll be our eyes, and watch us where we go
And help us to be wise, in times when we don't know
Let this be our prayer when we lose our way
Lead us to the place, guide us with your grace
To a place where we'll be safe.

I pray we'll find your light
And hold it in our hearts
When stars go out each night, let this be our prayer
When shadows fill our day, lead us to a place
Guide us with your grace.

Those who had heard it before had never listened to the words so closely. Everyone felt moved by the experience. Whenever I listen to it, it just picks my spirit up and holds it high. We all can use a good pick me up.

While relaxation-promoting music is perfect for the times you need to wind down, I found I also thrived on another form. While in treatment, I felt tired morning until night. I needed to be energized early in the day and at least stay up until mid-afternoon. Some days I was not seeing much purpose in getting out of bed and had to be convinced by my spirit that I should face the day upright. There's a magnetic property between pajamas/robes and sheets. Get clothes on – it helps. My chemotherapy started in December so I was right in the Christmas music season. The previous December I had fallen in love with "This is Your Gift." I played it every morning and let the CD run all day. This became my best way to energize, feel alive and appreciate the day in front of me.

This is Your Gift by John Tesh

If a *star can be a sign that the light is breaking through and a child*
      in your arms makes the whole world seem brand new-
We can embrace all the grace we've been given, stand in the light
      of the wonder we live in – This is your gift, this brand new day.

*So take it to heart, take it on faith. Open your eyes and don't be
    afraid to learn how to live cause this is your gift, this brand
    new day.*
*This is your gift when it's hard to say a prayer when you're over-
    come by fear and you see each day through a thousand falling
    tears.*
*Hope takes your hand, and it picks up the pieces. Love comes to
    life as we live and believe it.........*
*So take it to heart, take it on faith, open your eyes and don't be
    afraid to learn how to live*
*We'll take what God has given and live it from the heart – this is
    your gift.*

Some friends gave me wonderful gifts of CDs. Even loaning
some of your favorite music to a friend in need is a thoughtful way to
support them. Like sharing favorite books, music shared by friends
who know your taste is a treat.

AVAILABLE BODY & SPIRIT SUPPORTS

With every medical treatment, there is clinical evidence to prove each treatment has worked for some people. There's also evidence to prove it did not work for everyone. We need to appreciate we are unique individuals.

I felt the need to stay grounded with my medical team including oncologist, surgeon and the oncology nurses. I was most fortunate to have been diagnosed in a hospital that sponsors the position of Breast Care Center Coordinator. She contacted me immediately after my diagnosis and became my resource for all medically related questions. She was my security and stake in the ground as she helped me make decisions (by listening), located any information or data I requested, and best of all, became a friend. This nurse remained my primary source for informational support. She also directed me to complementary programs for and to other women who had a similar diagnosis past or present, giving me opportunity to learn from their experiences.

Cancer treatments and protocols for other major illnesses often go on for a long, long time. Time itself has a nasty habit of moving a lot slower when we don't feel well, compared to how quickly it flies when we are having fun. Based on the assumption you do not find treatment "fun", you know the anxiousness of trying to cope with how long it takes. I felt like a little kid asking over and over, "Are we there yet?" 'There' was the finish line – the end of treatment when I could turn the corner and start working ahead to recovery, return to full energy and normal life. Only later when I could look back did I realize progress was the greatest motivator during that stage. Progress can be measured in clicking off the days until the end of treatment, countdowns, recalculating the percentage of goal completed, etc. At the same time, I tried to celebrate having no delays or obstacles in the way. I even feared catching a computer virus! Note to care givers and visitors – sneezing within one mile of someone in countdown is forbidden.

Expectations I placed on myself and the expectations others put on me need to be balanced with the reality that it takes time to heal, recover and regain energy levels. Five weeks prior to my expected end date, I sent out invitations and planned my "coming back to life" party – Leap Year Eve, as it turned out. If you have not thought of celebrating – do it!

In an effort to adjust the medical treatments and the myriad of side effects from treatments, the non-pharmaceutical methods to enhance healing have inviting appeal.

FAITH SUPPORT

Faith support kept my spirit healthy and was the basis for all additional support and therapy in my recovery. If it were not for my spirit supporters nurturing my spirit every step of the way, my experience with cancer would have been much harder to bear and nothing but a struggle.

Active religious participation has documented benefits for improved health and over all well-being. A health crisis will kick these benefits into action. Dr. Levin describes three ways religious involvement will lead to support:

1. "Religious fellowship provides both tangible and emotional resources that buffer or reduce our experience of stress.
2. Active religious participation increases the likelihood that when stressful situations arise, they are put in a larger context

that offers greater meaning, and therefore is experienced less negatively.

3. Regular religious fellowship increases our access to people who can offer us assistance when we are in need – a network of friends in place." Levin pg. 60&61.

PRAYER

"The Lord didn't forget me, and He won't forget you. You have His awesome presence and His amazing grace. If you turn to Him in prayer, He will listen. If you seek Him with all your heart, you will find Him. He wants to give you a new beginning, a new purpose and renewed hope in the future. He wants to end your captivity and restore your prosperity. He wants to give you your life back…and He wants to be in the center." Nelson pg. 62

In addition to personal prayer, connect yourself to prayer ministries (see previous chapter).

ALPHA

Started in the 1990s, the program named Alpha has been attended by more than four million people all over the world. The Alpha program is an opportunity for anyone to explore the Christian faith in a relaxed, non-threatening setting. The ten weekly sessions are free of charge. It is supported by all the main Christian denominations. Alpha is offered primarily as an opportunity to explore the meaning of life to anyone who would like to attend. For further information and a listing of Alpha sessions near you, check their website at www.alphausa.org or www.alphacanada.org. I am thankful my parents took me to Sunday School and provided for my Christian upbringing and a solid foundation. Some of us have drifted away from the church and others are searching or have been disillusioned by organized Christianity. Alpha is worth considering. You will be in the company of others looking for life's answers.

EMOTIONAL AND SPIRITUAL SUPPORT

This form of support is the 'share a smoothie' type. Make an effort to keep the family and friends network informed of your progress and your emotional needs. We all need hugs. We also all need someone willing to listen to us vent when necessary. Pent- up emotions need release now more than ever. Stephen Ministry is the perfect combination of Christian spiritual and emotional support with trained listeners.

STEPHEN MINISTRY

The national, interdenominational Stephen Ministries have as their by-line, "Christ Caring for People through People." It is a one-to-one care giving ministry where God works through lay people (most are not clergy) to plant a seed of hope and healing in a person facing difficulty because of a life circumstance. Sometimes it helps to talk with someone who isn't family, not necessarily a close friend nor clergy or counselor. Lay people who have completed training to be Stephen Ministers are true listeners and encouragers. Congregations with this program offer support to members and non-members.

I have been trained to be a Stephen Minister. Needless to say, I had my contacts in place although I never expected to be the care-receiver. It's very true that there is a limit to how much you want to burden your family emotionally. A Stephen Minister will bring an uninvolved perspective that is still full of caring. A person to pray with you and be there to help steady you on the Christian path is a wonderful gift. It is worth exploring or asking a Christian friend to see if a program is near you and make the connection. You will have a new friend, too.

TANGIBLE SUPPORTS

A ministry in my home church is called 'Love Your Neighbor'. This is a group of volunteers who offer many services. Some give rides to appointments, some prepare and deliver meals, others run errands, help with basic chores, baby-sit, etc. A couple of people coordinate the requests or needs and match them up with a volunteer. It's a wonderful service that makes the connection between those offering to give some Christian love in hands and feet service to others who need the support. I was blessed to be a recipient of this ministry.

New in 2004, *Lotsa Helping Hands When Friends & Family Need Help,* was set up on a website, www.lotsahelpinghands.com. It demonstrates a "simple, immediate way for friends, family, colleagues and neighbors to assist loved ones in need. It's an easy to use, private group calendar, specifically designed for organizing helpers." Wonderful, innovative and practical 'helps' keep coming out. How fortunate for us in need.

At the same time, family, friends and neighbors knew I would have needs and also knew I would be reluctant to ask for help. Some of the best support is the call where a loving, assertive voice says, "I'm bringing you and your husband dinner on Friday night. Is 6 p.m. okay?"

Susan lives across the street from me and detests shopping. I'm sure she has her reasons. Starting my chemotherapy in December, she offered to do my Christmas shopping for me on condition that I gave her a list. What a gift!

I was amazed at the resourcefulness and creative offers of help I received. Tangible support is wonderful. Be willing to accept this support. In the future, you will be able to pass on the love by volunteering or taking some leadership to organize a similar service.

SUPPORT GROUPS

Especially for breast cancer, but also many other cancers and diseases, support groups have been set up at health care facilities, churches and community centers. Benefits vary from person to person and group to group. Many women cannot imagine having breast cancer without their support group and have made treasured, life long friends. Others never find the right mix of group members and some prefer other forms of support.

Before joining a group, be realistic in how much time and energy you can devote to attending a group and how far you really want to travel to meet with them. Some groups meet less often than others do.

Most groups will have a facilitator or a contact person. Susan G. Komen Foundation affiliates will provide you a list to call as will the American Cancer Society. Before visiting, spend time calling the facilitator and get a feel for the group. You may not want to be the only one in your 30's while all the other members are of retirement age. Your comfort level in the group may be better when at least some of the members are also fairly newly diagnosed.

In general, treatments for cancer go on for months and there is tremendous benefit in being with others who have "been there done that." Being able to share what has worked well or made the treatment easier to live with is valuable information. Also, making the connection with others who totally understand your feelings and your fears is comforting. Encouragement from those with this level of true understanding is marvelous.

Explore what class offerings may be available through your clinic or community if this is your first experience with a major or chronic illness. I think of such classes as an orientation. They can calm fears and are the best exposure to what services and supports are locally available to you. Usually family and/or friends may also attend. This will help care-givers and supporters feel comfortable in their new roles and provide resources to them.

Separate groups are frequently set up for those who have had cancer at least once before. The direction of these groups is to affirm life and share insights of emotional strength as all are experienced and have earned advanced degrees in coping.

Dr. David Spiegel of Stanford University School of Medicine has shown the value of group therapy in three important ways. First, a support group will build bonds by preventing social isolation and providing an outlet for the 'helper therapy principle' (you help your-self by helping others). Secondly, the group encourages the expression of emotion to face feelings directly. In a group, you can be upset, you can cry, release the emotion and prepare to move forward. And third, by facing the serious issues with others, we can detoxify dying, lessen the anxiety and move beyond the fear that we can not handle it. In studies done by Dr. Spiegel, those who participated in a support group outlived those who did not join a group.

In my own situation, I was not able to find a local support group with a schedule that worked for me. A mutual friend told Cathy, who lived only a half mile from me, that I had been diagnosed within days of her diagnosis. Cathy invited me out for coffee and we became a group of two. She was ten days ahead of me on the same chemotherapy drugs. Our conversations could jump right to the center of our concerns. Having cancer together, with ability to both share and understand the other's needs, created the best friendship bond. We celebrated every step of progress such as the completion of each chemo treatment, end of all treatment, first good check up, recovery, hair (well, fuzz) return, first day without a wig, first haircut, one year anniversary, etc. CELEBRATE EVERY LITTLE THING YOU CAN! – Cathy and I swear by it!

SUPPORT SUMMARY

All supports mentioned really complement each other. As we go through life, we support each other in many ways. With a health crisis to manage, your family and friends will come out and rally for you as you would for them. Ask for and accept this support by considering it acts of Christian love. There is no reason to turn it down.

COMPLEMENTARY THERAPIES

Many of the lists readily available for complementary/alternative cures suggest that through various approaches, you have the power to heal yourself using methods of mind and body control. Be wary of pagan spirituality based on far-fetched imaginations. Lofty speculations easily get in the way of seeing the true and living God standing close by waiting to be called upon. You will not be alone to stick exclusively with the Lord as your sure comforter and healer. Choosing to avoid distraction can be your choice.

"For this people's heart has become calloused; they hardly hear with their ears, and they have closed their eyes. Otherwise they might see with their eyes, hear with their ears, understand with their hearts and turn, and I (Jesus) would heal them." Matthew 13:15 NIV

If we make our choices based on worldly philosophies or healing techniques, we become blind and deaf to the spiritual messages God is sending. Many times I felt it was so easy to be led astray. Satan is always at work. Prayer and awareness of God's signs light our path. We will know which choices to make by keeping our eyes and ears sharp to recognize truth over confusion.

It is the Lord who will heal you according to His plan for you. I believe it is God's expectation that we avail ourselves to medical technology and be responsible in caring for our human body. God gave you the intellect to follow your doctor's orders, take the prescribed medications and choose between recommended treatment options. Apart from God, there is nothing you can do yourself to change His plan or heal yourself. God alone will do it.

Past the initial shock, I think we tend to be more open and receptive to exploring what complementary therapies are available to make the process easier, more manageable or more comfortable. Others have gone before us and have helped to develop and expand a number of complementary opportunities. Any physical comfort that comes to a sick, tired body will help you cope and will ease stress. If you are receiving Western medicine treatment, some following therapies, which originated in Eastern medicine, would be considered complementary versus alternative to Western medicine. Some programs may help by lessening physical discomfort and some may not. Discontinue attending any program that hints or boldly feels contrary to your faith in the Lord.

AROMATHERAPY

This is the therapeutic use of essential oils from flowers, leaves, roots and stems. Aromas are either inhaled or applied to the skin. Be wary of oils that may be ingested as there are no guidelines for how they will interact with medications. Many of the chemotherapy drugs cause a heightened sense of smell. Aromatherapy that is soothing and helps to bring on a relaxed feeling can be wonderful gifts. Scented candles, lavender bath oils and jasmine lotion, etc. all may pamper a body that by day is poked and prodded for medical reasons and needs relief in the evening. A warm, long bath before slipping into bed may take away the tension of the day and help you sleep. If relaxing aromas enhance this, go ahead and pamper.

Before my biopsy, I was treated to a student experimenting with rubbing oils on my arms to calm me. By measuring my blood pressure before and after, this clinically showed a positive response. I did not need the data to know I had less anxiety – it was wonderful. Many more applications of aromatherapy will be commonly used as this technique advances.

ACUPUNCTURE

Needles are placed at the acupoints (365 specific points in the body) to stimulate and remove energy blockages. The theory is that pain and nausea can be relieved, circulation improved, tension and stress eased, immune function enhanced, blood pressure lowered and improved sleeping patterns will result. Skin is a barrier to sources of infection and acupuncture does break that barrier. If taking prescribed anti-coagulants, there may be a risk.

Of the people I know who have tried acupuncture, half thought it was of benefit and half did not. I have no personal experience, but really feel that someone who is currently in treatment and has not tried this method before their illness should probably wait to try it once back on the recovery side.

LOOK GOOD....FEEL BETTER

This is a "free, non-medical, brand-neutral, national public service program founded in 1989 and supported by corporate donors to help women offset appearance related changes from cancer treatment." Learning a few beauty techniques and ways to combat the side effects of dry skin and hair loss did help me to look better and I felt better. It's a wonderful service. There is a mail order video available if no program is close enough for you to attend. Programs are also available in Spanish and for teens with cancer. Check www. lookgoodfeelbetter.org for more information and treat yourself.

MASSAGE

Types of massage vary and not all are appropriate during cancer treatment.

Swedish style massage with vigorous strokes and kneading of the muscles is better for a body that's fully healthy. My basic rule was that if the massage was a great work out for the person giving the massage, it is best saved for healthier days. More desirable is a massage that is gentle and will enhance physical and psychological relaxation.

Shiatsu massage comes from Japanese tradition and uses pressure points to release energy blockages within the energy system of the body. I tried the massage only once when I was having a really bad day. I couldn't feel the full benefit as I was not allowing it to relax me, or maybe I was just blocking it out. **Acupressure** (Chinese) is similar.

Healing Touch Massage was offered free to those in chemotherapy at the breast care center from a generous donor. Healing Touch is not intended to be curative, but rather complements conventional medical care. There is very little touch and the process is aided with relaxation music in the background. By working with the energy field over your body, they are able to bring the feeling of relaxation and balance in a peaceful state. I admit to being a bit of a skeptic, however after 45 minutes of this very gentle massage, I was totally relaxed. When I stood up I felt like my feet were as padded as baby's feet. The massage let me release all the low-grade pains and discomforts of the side effects of chemotherapy. Give yourself permission to physically feel better and psychologically you will smile all the way home.

GUIDED IMAGERY

"Guided imagery is a process of deliberately using your imagination to help your mind and body heal, stay well or perform well. It's a kind of directed, deliberate daydream, a purposeful creation of positive sensory images – sights, sounds, smells, tastes and feel – in your imagination. For example, you might create images of your immune cells fighting germs or of your pulse rate slowing down; you might recall in exacting sensory detail an absent loved one for extra emotional comfort; or you could "rehearse" a perfect golf swing moments before you actually heft your club. Under the right conditions, your mind and body will believe these images are real, and will respond accordingly, with varying degrees of efficiency, intensity, and success." Naperstek p. 198.

One-on-one or in a small group, imagery allows you to have healing images control the personal feelings about cancer or other disease. For imagery to work, you must be in a relaxed, focused state. While possible to learn on your own, I found that having a trained practitioner teach me how to be receptive to the imagery process was very beneficial. Guided imagery typically leads you to have a mental guide (you can choose the guide such as the Holy Spirit, a parent, a grandparent, a favorite teacher). Choose one you can confide in with ease. I felt tremendous strength to see and feel in my mind the Holy Spirit walking down a path with me offering guidance all the way. Personally, I benefited tremendously from imagery and guided imagery.

Bellaruth Naperstek's book is a good introductory resource. Her website at www.healthjourneys.com offers books and CDs for imagery including ones specific for cancer, heart disease, sleep relaxation and others.

The Academy for Guided Imagery at www.academyforguided-imagery.com states their purpose is to help or guide people to being active in their own healing process. At their website, they will direct you to a trained practitioner in your area.

AFFIRMATIONS

Similar to guided imagery, listening to and then repeating in your mind affirmations that you are healing, you have hope, etc. are very positive energy generators. B. Naperstek offers CDs that have both guided imagery and affirmations. She has commented in her books that she's received the most positive responses on the last affirmation on her CDs where she helps listeners to visualize and accept they are safe in God's hands. I know my body reacted positively to hearing that it was safe and the affirmation made my healthy spirit happy.

MEDITATION AND SEEKING TRUTH

While traveling on the treatment path, it's normal to feel power-less. Dependence is placed on the medical professionals to manage all the medical pieces for us, and in the face of fatigue, we may expect our family and prayer friends to take care of our mental and spiritual support needs. We still need to participate in our own healing and do what we can to make the journey as pleasant as possible. Our spirit offers up the strength to help our bodies heal. We can overcome our feelings of powerlessness by learning to connect with our spirit which will help us to feel secure.

Pope Benedict XVI has made statements addressing his concern that the Christian moral foundations are being threatened in our society. No prayers in schools, the removal of the Ten Commandments from public buildings, and other attempts to keep God in the background or completely out of the picture may produce a society led by the moral standards of governments and individuals. "It's telling that the final draft of the European constitution left God out of its preamble. According to the most recent European Values Study, just 21 percent of Europeans say religion is very important to them. A Gallup poll last year (2004) found that on average only about 15 percent of Europe's people attend a place of worship once a week, compared with 44 percent of Americans." C. Dickey. These statistics point out that there are many alternatives to the Christian faith and clearly they have a draw. In desperate search for comfort and peace of mind, we seek and are curious to find solace and relief from the inevitable stress of dealing with a health crisis day after day. Long treatment plans and the lengthy wait of knowing if the treatment will be successful stress our psyches beyond a quick fix medical problem.

"The pagan high places of today are many and varied, but they are nothing new. They include such lofty speculations as higher consciousness, crystals, karma, reincarnation...and they promote strains of native mysticism, universal forces or energies and higher powers (masters)." Weber p.197. An endless supply of self-help books and teachings of New Age philosophies are readily available. We live in an age where many hear just what they want to hear from their religious background (or lack of) and by giving it a slight twist, they can custom make their own form of religion. Those with the gift of leadership then capably lead others to follow them in their new philosophies/religion. Creating a religion adjusted to fit a person's own comfort level is not God's plan.

"...I (Jesus) am the way and the truth and the life. No one comes to the Father except through me." John 14:6 NIV

Does truth become whatever you want it to be – whatever serves your interests in the moment? Some have constructed truth and made it up for themselves, like the ultimate do-it-yourself project. When "everything is relative," it becomes a matter of perspective or how you choose to see things. It is easy to get buried in one perspective that ultimately matters – your own. However, what is true for you may not be true for others. So if we can get ourselves to the core of the universe with self-talk, self-renewal, our own unique energy source and presumed guide we will successfully cloud reality. In this search for truth, the seeker will be deterred or at least delayed in grasping the reality of God who is standing by waiting to be called upon.

"It is better to depend on the Lord than to trust mortals." Psalm 118:8 (God's Word)

In some ways, others views may prevent you from receiving grace inspired insights. Checking out other's views has its place, as long as these views do not get in the way of our own inner spiritual guidance.

"I can do everything through Christ who strengthens me." Philippians 4:13 (God's Word)

Meditation is a kind of mental retreat to strengthen your connection to God via spirituality. It centers around breathing and focusing the mind on the present moment. It allows individuals to experience the limitless nature of the mind when it ceases to be dominated by its usual mental chatter. Meditation is used to balance a person's physical, emotional and mental states and is an aid in treating stress, pain, heart disease and other conditions. Meditation allows the individual to listen to his or her spirit to make the best personal choices.

Dr. Benson refers to the "relaxation response" to manage stress and maintain wellness. We so often try to listen over the noise of life. Silence is good self-care. When we calm the mind, we flood the body with health-enhancing chemicals and gain access to important information about who we are, how we feel, and what we need.

Complementary therapies are available and allow you to focus on healing, decrease tension and help maintain inner peace. Being more relaxed and less directed by fears encourages your body to heal and restore itself.

In meditation, we lock minds in the present and thus free ourselves from worries of the past or fears of the future. There is a sense of peace and confidence that all is moving in the right direction and according to God's plan. Meditation can help us to really focus on developing a strong bond with our spirit. It will make surrendering to the guidance of the spirit more natural and desirable. Spirit transcends time and space, offering the peaceful flow of life in the big picture.

Common meditation practices are Yoga, Qigong, and Tai Chi. All three of these techniques are based on self-awareness, well-being, and energy flow through the body. The basis is that the body's vital energy force needs to be cultivated. The exercises are gentle motions designed to move the energy force gently through your body. These exercises are sometimes done in preparation for meditation and are all from Eastern healing traditions. None are based on Christianity, however.

The goal of common forms of meditation is to bring about altered states of consciousness bordering on mystical or paranormal for some. Dr. Jeff Levin summarizes his extensive studies on this topic as follows: "I found that these experiences were reported more frequently by people who were more privately and subjectively religious, but less frequently by people who participate in organized religion, even after controlling for things like age, sex, ethnicity, socioeconomic status, and other dimensions of religiousness. The conclusion was unavoidable: institutional religion apparently discourages or depresses the experience of mystical states of consciousness." Levin pg. 157. He further describes the phenomenology of altered states of consciousness and the associated energies or forces to be "accepted by some scientists, rejected by others, held to be delusions by some clinicians, and the source of varying degrees of apprehension among traditionally religious people." Levin pg. 163.

Meditation is what a person makes it. Prayer is a form of meditation. Christians will use a centering prayer while meditating to maintain their focus. In general we think of prayer as talking with or to God. Centering prayer differs in that it is a way to silence your mind to be fully present so you can listen to the wisdom of God within. First, choose a sacred word or phrase to use as a symbol of your intention to invite the Holy Spirit to be within you. Examples might be: Father, Abba, Lord, Jesus, peace, or mercy. Next, position yourself so you are comfortable with eyes closed and begin introducing your sacred word to your silence. Remain in silence. Allow your mind to be fully present and listen for God's wisdom to speak to you.

I found the whole package for meditation and mind peace (the peace that passes all understanding) in the truths of Christianity. I needed help to feel I was keeping my spirit healthy and recognized it was way beyond my control. It worked for me to integrate my spiritual strength and my spirit's wisdom. It takes effort and courage to reach out and explore. Rely on your spirit to guide you to these choices and have confidence in the spirit directing you. Should you feel a drift too far from the Lord or the focus of your meditation becomes a master other than Christ, trust that your spirit will give you the courage to leave behind what you do not believe in or what creates conflict in your mind. At times, I felt unsettled and quit when getting too close to depending on my own energy force like a form of mystical magic.

"Be strong, all who wait with hope for the Lord, and let your heart be courageous." Psalm 31:24 (God's Word)

POTHOLES ON THE PATH

"Even youths grow tired and weary, and young men stumble and fall: but those who hope in the Lord will renew their strength. They will soar on wings like eagles; they will run and not grow weary, they will walk and not be faint." Isaiah 40:30-31. NIV

In the ideal world, every path would be a smooth one. For two to three months, early each spring in Minnesota we engage in something called Pothole Season where the pavement gets sinkholes from the freezing and thawing action below the road's surface. It drives our visitors crazy dodging them, but a good Minnesotan artfully drives around them and patiently waits out the end of frost. Maybe we just know the end is in sight and there is nothing to do other than continue down the road. Our employers expect we will figure it out and get to work even if there has been a detour along our path.

"In every way we're troubled, but we aren't crushed by our troubles. We're frustrated, but we don't give up." 2 Corinthians 4:8 (God's Word)

Along the path of treatment for an illness, potholes will inevitably appear. Some people refer to these as 'setbacks'. A 'setback' is full of negative connotations and often closes our minds to a pothole that could be an opportunity in disguise. What is hard is to see is that an unexpected change can often be good when it happens. In the big picture, when we take a blind swan dive into a pothole, what can we do but climb out and keep going? Of course, the sooner we crawl out, the better. Jesus is standing nearby waiting to be asked to nudge, lift, drag or carry you out of the hole – whatever it takes, He will get you out as soon as you reach out to Him.

"The Lord will be your confidence. He will keep your foot from getting caught." Proverbs 3:26 (God's Word)

I had completed the necessary surgeries and preparation to start chemotherapy. Suddenly, I felt compelled to question my physician if he was totally confident my breast cancer had not already spread to the other side. It was a strange feeling as the Holy Spirit encouraged my spirit to question my doctor. Bluntly spoken, the words surprised me. I will never know if another doctor would have taken my concern seriously as it was such a long shot. However, my doctor promptly ordered a PET scan. The same day that I was to start chemotherapy was the day my test results came back. My doctor, bless his heart, has body language that is very easy to interpret. The shock hit me full strength before he finished his clinical explanations. He told me a second, independent cancer had started and I would need to go back to surgery before starting on chemo. What a pothole that was! The stun gun all over again. For this to happen was clinically next to impossible, and I have heard that my films made the rounds all over the Twin Cities area at a number of radiologist's conferences. Maybe I'm due a royalty.

If I had chosen to ignore my spirit's prompting to ask about my far-fetched concern, the consequence would have been unsuccessful treatment, discovery of the second cancer much later, with a greater challenge to control and stop it. Another piece of God's Plan for me was revealed that day. I knew I would survive and was all the more reassured the Lord was keeping my spirit healthy. It was a gift of grace that I heard the prompting of the Holy Spirit within me. So, Jesus wasted no time getting me up and out of the pothole, nudged me to be proactive, do the surgery (the detour) and get back to the treatment path. I knew I was supposed to keep going until I reached the finish line. It was only possible for me to be positive about this setback as I was so clearly feeling guidance and direction.

Once we are deep into a major illness that we clearly did not ask for, we can choose to be better for the experience OR be bitter and allow the negative to dominate. The experience of having cancer certainly helped me to grow in faith and I am not bitter – I'm better for it. The path may well be long and God's Plan for you may include a few potholes. Keep your spirit healthy and hang on tightly to your faith in God and His gifts of grace and guidance.

"You, too, must be patient. Don't give up hope..." James 5:8 (God's Word)

BIG POTHOLES

With treatment comes side effects that are certainly potholes along the path for many of us. Fortunately, most of us get just some, not all, of the possible side effects. The best advice is to keep your doctor informed when any potential side effect is causing you concern or discomfort. We are all unique and will react uniquely to treatments.

SLEEP DEPRIVATION

Nothing kept me crawling on gravel my entire path more than sleep deprivation. It can take down the happiest of happy, positive people. We have to just give in to allowing our bodies the rest and sleep they need to heal and recover. In my case, I had some drug interactions with medications outside of cancer treatment that prevented me from sleeping which left me 'wired' and awake up to twenty hours a day. We all are different and I sure do not wish my drug sensitivities on anyone. Fatigue caused by lack of sleep makes coping much harder. Be sure your physician is aware if sleep is limited. Be kind to yourself and cut back on your work schedule, recognize your reflexes may be less than optimal for driving safely and know it is all normal. Sit with any group of survivors and most will admit they regret they had not cut back work and activities farther and made fewer commitments when their bodies were begging for 'down time' to heal and recover.

CHEMO BRAIN

It's a charming name, but again a very common side effect. When you start to think making a grocery list is too big a challenge, it might be. So let it be one more thing to delegate. The good news here is that it is temporary and happens later in treatment so it won't last long. Be kind to yourself and think positively. With chemo brain, I was still able to hear my spirit and it quite possibly my mind was cleared from worries I didn't need.

"So don't ever worry about tomorrow. After all, tomorrow will worry about itself. Each day has enough trouble of its own." Matthew 6:34 (God's Word)

FATIGUE

"He gives power to the tired and worn out, and strength to the weak." Isaiah 40:29 (TLB)

Some people are fortunate to dodge most of the other side effects, but, fatigue will hit virtually everyone in both chemotherapy and radiation treatment. It is nature's way of slowing us down and letting the cells repair themselves and heal. Depending on the extent, there are all sorts of ways to conserve your energy. It is hard to give up activities in the name of energy conservation, but again, remember, it's temporary. I sat in the clinic one visit whining to my doctor I was so fatigued that I couldn't even do a half mile on my treadmill. He responded, "Put it away." I know I'll never hear that advice again; he made my day.

"That is why we are not discouraged. Though outwardly we are wearing out, inwardly we are renewed day by day." 2 Corinthians 4:16 (God's Word)

DEPRESSION

Depression is a serious condition that can further complicate a patient's journey to wellness. It can be the result of long buried emotional pain that is triggered by stresses on the job, health issues, financial pressures, grief, etc. One day we're happily bouncing thru life and the next we have a life threatening diagnosis = STRESS. For most, an illness will not be the one and only exclusive stress. The day before my cancer diagnosis, my husband and I were leading lives that included stress. My personal health crisis tipped the scale to depression.

"God allowed some of the greatest people of faith to remain in depression for years." (Weber p. 232).

Laughter and humor are marvelous antidotes to counteract mild depression. For the women who do look spectacular bald, they may well miss out on the wig humor. My husband and I go out with two other couples every month to different restaurants as unpaid but experienced food critics of sorts. When I was unable to go out, they came to us and brought dinner with them. Our group always has a fun time and we love to laugh at stupid stuff. These cheerleaders brought to me a piece of normal life which eased my isolation, great food and best of all, a few laughs. During the long haul, they made sure I got a dose of needed laughter often. I noticed that the mood of greeting cards I received changed also. More serious cards in the beginning gradually gave way to the funny "get well" cards intended to offer me a little chuckle. My friend, Heidi, knew I was hard-up for entertainment and sent me a child's dot to dot card. Cheerleaders are priceless, and I would have sunk much deeper without them.

"A joyful heart is good medicine, but depression drains one's strength." Proverbs 17:22 (God's Word)

Sleep deprivation, fatigue and any of the treatment side effects compound to fuel depression. There are many levels of depression, from mild to extreme. Clinical depression can and will disrupt your life. The literature listing the potential side effects of some of the chemotherapy drugs include "depression." Chemical imbalances, drug interactions and blatant side effects of some drugs can cause depression.

Get help. Get help. Get help.

For those of us raised to be stoic and/or to resist seeking professional mental health counseling, getting help becomes a bit of a struggle. When the stresses of cancer, normal life, sleep deprivation, chemo side effects, and lack of energy all came together, I sought professional help. If depression is untreated, it will only slow your recovery. Care-givers and those living in the same house need to watch carefully for potential depression and may need to initiate getting professional help. As we breeze in and out of a doctor's office, there is lab work and all the medical business to divert attention from the signs of depression. I successfully hid my depression at doctor appointments or so I believed. It is no surprise that we, the victims of depression, will be the last to bring it up or to seek help, as we are busy covering depression from view. It is critical for care-givers to listen, to watch for signs and symptoms and to be proactive by encouraging professional assistance.

"He is the healer of the brokenhearted. He is the one who bandages their wounds." Psalm 147:3 (God's Word)

THE FINAL STRETCH

Hold the Big Picture in front of you. Each day feels like a slow crawl down a path that seems endless. Your goal is to get to the end of treatment and cross the finish line. Hopefully your cheerleaders are checking in with you regularly to help keep your vision clear as the goal comes closer. Trust that God through his grace will show you the path.

"I can do everything through Christ who strengthens me."
Philippians 4:13(God's Word)

Knowing that people around us care, helps nurture the healing process. How cooperative we are will also make all the difference in the world.

"I've learned that even when I have pains, I don't have to be one." Maya Angelou

It's hard to imagine that as late as the early 1960s, people still were able to check themselves into an American hospital for a week of R&R – rest and relaxation. Now we have spas or other options for retreats for basic R&R. I have thought it would be fun to stop in at a hospital admitting office and ask if they offer an all-inclusive five-day R&R package.

Hospital in-patients today are sick, injured or recovering from some health adversity. With cost containment practices, rapidly changing technology and regulations for maintaining records, etc., hospital employees have very demanding jobs. Just at the time their patients have their pain controlled, feel a little better and become more pleasant to be around, they are discharged and a new really sick patient rolls into the room.

A tiny bit of appreciation expressed to these hard-working hospital staff goes a long, long way. You don't have to be a pain. At a minimum, THANK YOU is easy enough and always appreciated. Individually wrapped chocolates, the ultimate comfort food to share with the hospital staff are a nice touch. My daughter who is a certified orthotist and visits 3-5 hospital patients daily brought my chocolate supply to the hospital for me. Her recommendation is one bag per day and even greater appreciation can be expressed by giving a choice between two varieties. A few staff have turned me down due to allergies, but were glad to tuck a few candies into their pocket to take home or share at coffee breaks. Be sure to give the housekeeping staff chocolate when they enter the room. I know I had the cleanest room! An appreciative, chocolate loving happy lab tech was the person I wanted to do my blood draws.

Another way to show basic courtesy and not be a pain is to call hospital staff by their names. This is especially true of the ones who will be around you all day. To say, "Thank You, Barb, for taking care of me all night" holds a lot more weight than just "Thanks." It's a personal connection and it helps them feel good about the job they did that day or night. We all are energized knowing our care, our effort or our specialized training was put to good use. Barb's dedication may well have been kicked up a notch.

On the third day of a post-surgery hospital stay, a nurse who had been there every day on the day shift came in my room and started up a chat. After 15 minutes of delightful, non-medical conversation I had to wonder if I was there for R&R after all. I couldn't help but finally ask him how he had so much free time that day as typically he moved just short of a jog from room to room. He told me he chose to take his afternoon break in my room as he thought I was fun to talk to. I didn't have any pain while my nurse posed as a visitor and I enjoyed a refreshing escape from the reality of why I was in a hospital bed. Certainly my confidence level went up and I felt much more secure in his care. By the way, this nurse didn't care for chocolate.

"I've learned that no matter what happens, or how bad it seems today, life does go on, and it will be better tomorrow." Maya Angelou

When the long treatment path seems endless, the desperation point (some would say the "turning point"), is where we are most apt to turn to God. The ability to surrender is a sign of spiritual maturity. It can be the realization that we actually are not in control no matter how much we wish we were. It is not our spirits trying to control and direct our lives, it is our egos. Without a doubt, we want and like to do it all our own way. When we are finally ready to listen, look for the signs and be open. God never left you. You merely freed-up what was there all along, the Light of God. Now you can stop trying to figure it all out on your own. Believing God has a plan for your life allows you the freedom to let go and trust God to manage your well-being today and the future. "If you don't learn to surrender your will, you will surrender your peace." Richardson pg. 141. Acceptance, trust and surrender opens the door to show us the way. God has promised that he will carry our burdens for us, if only we let Him.

"Cast all your anxiety on him because he cares for you." 1 Peter 5:7 NIV

Cheryl Richardson's book, <u>The Unmistakable Touch of Grace</u> was very inspiring to me. Many things or events happen in our lives and we so easily write them off to 'coincidences'. When we open our eyes and hearts to the possibility, we realize many "coincidences" are really acts of God's grace. Staying connected to God thru our spirits offers us our best chance to survive and be well in our challenging world. Every crisis of our lives is another step toward spiritual wholeness and one we share with supportive Christians. During those times we may question our faith or forget to surrender our will, but having Christians 'on call' will help steer us back. We sometimes need help remembering God is the ultimate support for all of us. It is through God's grace the light on the path continues to shine.

"You saved me from death. You saved my eyes from tears (and) my feet from stumbling." Psalm 116:8 (God's Word)

"Every day we receive, and offer others gifts of grace. Once you see how people are planting seeds for your spiritual growth, either through the support they give you, or the challenges they present, every conversation you have becomes so much more than just an exchange of thoughts or ideas. It becomes a communion of sorts; a sacred event that, in some way big or small, has the power to change you forever." Richardson pg. 122. What on the surface appeared to be a chance meeting or someone new walking into your life may be an act of grace.

"...taking immediate action is another important conduit for receiving the gift of grace. The more time we waste analyzing our moves, considering the negative consequences of our actions, or thinking about our fear, the greater the possibility that we'll interrupt the flow of thoughts, feeling and ideas that we most want and need to express." Richardson pg. 115.

Huge decisions must be made carefully. When you have been guided by grace to take a step and move on it, stalling may only result in talking yourself into indecision. Many times I felt at crossroads for making decisions in regard to surgery options and treatment choices. It was a gift of grace to feel the guidance of my spirit replacing indecision, with arrows and light indicating the right path. With peace of mind, a tremendous gift itself, I could go forward and stay on that long path.

END OF TREATMENT

The long road of treatment finally ends. *CELEBRATE!!*

"He restores my soul; He leads me in the paths of righteousness for His name's sake." Psalm 23:3 NIV

The key word for me in this verse is ***restores***. There is no covering-up a traumatic experience (I'm still *not* calling it a "battle") with a major illness which rocked us with fear and insecurity did not happen – it did. Rather, we have the promise that we will be restored. The detours have ended. As God restores our energy, hopes, and health, our spirits will also be restored and rejoicing.

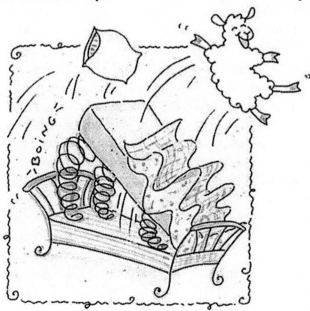

Be kind to yourself and give yourself time to heal. It would be great if all your strength and energy returned overnight. To be realistic, take it easy and ease your way back. I got the treadmill back out which was both bad and good. I was appalled at how little strength and stamina I had after treatment. But, with the treadmill, I could see from the numbers on the screen that I was walking longer and faster each day. Progress will motivate, as will cheerleaders. Literally, it took me months to achieve a full mile on the treadmill. Friends cheered and congratulated me. Every person is different as are our reactions to treatment. I suggest being conservative on your expectations of how quickly your energy will return. Family, be realistic about your survivor's energy level before zipping off on a vacation. If short on stamina, travel may not be the fun you had hoped for and it may be a better idea a few months later.

Typically, after treatment ends, there is a re-assessment period where tests are run to assure that treatment has stopped the cancer. The focus will shift to managing the risks and all forms of prevention available. Having the knowledge of what you as a unique individual can do for prevention will mean decisions and choices. Genetic studies for a number of cancers are advancing rapidly. We are on the horizon of tapping into the mysteries on many genetic fronts for many diseases. If you are not the first in your bloodline to have cancer, take advantage of genetic counseling and determine if genetic testing is appropriate for you. To have what is commonly called a cancer gene means an individual has less than normal defenses against cancer starting and therefore is at a higher risk than the average person is. To know you are at higher risk gives family members (no, not spouses) the information they need to consider testing. Should a cancer gene be present which is uncommon in the general population, numerous opportunities for prevention and early detection become possible.

With the end of treatment, a refreshed feeling of restored control comes back. Again, let your spirit be your guide for the best prevention path for you to follow. Peace of mind is attainable even with the knowledge and awareness of the risks that the disease could return.

REMISSION

For decades, 'remission' was the common term used when someone completed cancer treatment and no evidence of the cancer could be detected in the blood or by scans. As we survivors rejoin the world and resume normal activities, it seems an all-too-easy term to explain away our current condition. This is a term we need to eliminate from our cancer dictionary! It infers that cancer cells are hiding out somewhere in our body anxiously awaiting the opportunity to cluster and start a new tumor. Those of us who have had cancer know that we are not just temporarily out of the active state of the disease; we are cancer free and should be celebrating our health and well-being. At the same time, we know we are at risk for seeing cancer again.

It's pure anxiety to live with the fear and to hear the term 'remission'. Those fears stir up negative emotions. When I was asked if I was in remission, my answer was always, "No. I don't have cancer anymore." How you perceive your current health status will reflect, outwardly, how you want others to relate to you. Supporters are looking for your cues, so give them! Another way to phrase it would be, "Instead of remission, a more empowering and playful expression might be, 'I have transcended the diagnosis!' or 'I moved right past remission and on to perfect health." Chiappone pg. 283.

Physicians today suggest a much more aggressive and frequent follow-up plan, including more frequent check-ups for any sign of a cancer's return. At times I felt the rope was too short, but I loved the confidence gained from the frequent checks. When treatment ends, the 'All Clear' is given. That is exactly what it is. All clear, no detectable cells on the loose, no need for treatment, no cancer cells hiding, it's over, done – move on.

Prior to 2001, limited research was available for the long-term issues for adult survivors. Long-term follow-up care clinics for survivors of childhood cancers do exist. Grants from the Susan G. Komen Foundation and the Lance Armstrong Foundation have resulted in more focus and availability for adult survivors. Check the 'Progress' section on Lance Armstrong Foundation website at www.laf.org for the latest updates. With these grants and increased interest secondary to increasing numbers of long-term cancer survivors, in 2005, Centers for Disease Control and Prevention created *A National Action Plan for Cancer Survivorship: Advancing Public Health Strategies.* "It was developed to identify and prioritize cancer survivorship needs and strategies within the context of public health that will ultimately improve the overall experience and quality of life of the millions of Americans who are living with, through, and beyond cancer." Pg.12.

SANDPLAY

I was privileged to participate in Dr. Dale Ellen Grossman's new program of Sandplay for breast cancer survivors. She and some of her colleagues are working to bring this therapy into more common practice. It really helped me transition from treatment into recovery and the survivor mentality.

"Sandplay is a non-verbal technique in which miniature figures are used symbolically in the sand. The manipulation of the sand combined with the creativity of the play allows for a healing experience. Sandplay has been compared to a 'waking dream' as well as to a 'meditation with symbols'. No interpretation is given at the time of the sandplay, however, a deep knowing is frequently experienced by the sandplayer. Photos are taken of the trays and viewed two months after the last tray. At this meeting, interpretations may be shared.

The diagnosis and treatment of breast cancer is a life-changing event. The woman who emerges from treatment is different than the person who existed prior to diagnosis: physically, spiritually and emotionally. Sandplay provides one way to process and give form to this transformation." Dr. Grossman.

BEING A SURVIVOR

Upon being declared a survivor, there is a feeling of guilt for many which is probably rooted in unresolved grief for those who did not achieve survivor status. Accept that healing is a process and that God's plan for you remains steady and sure.

Recovery stirs pride and punctuates the new identity of being a survivor. It's time to celebrate again. The Susan G. Komen Foundation Race for the Cure annual Mother's Day event was a perfect way for me to wear the survivor's pink shirt and participate with my family. With the event as a goal (to be able to walk--only my daughter actually ran) helped my treadmill efforts. It is a great way to raise funds for the foundation and cancer research. I volunteer in a third grade classroom and included the children to be supporters also. I fashioned paper pompoms with pink and white streamers and asked the children to be my cheerleaders by each signing a streamer for me as did all my supporters and medical staff whether they financially contributed or not. My pompoms were the envy of everyone. It was fun and the adults loved it as much as the kids did.

Cathy, the other half of my support group, and I went to HealthEast Foundation's (St. Paul, MN) annual women cancer survivor's conference which was during the week of our first anniversary of diagnosis. We were both in awe of how wonderful it felt to be in such good company. Not short on words, we reported back how special we thought the conference was. A few months later we were contacted as representative attendees to help with the promotion of the next year's conference by writing a letter to sponsors. It was another way we felt we could benefit others by being survivors.

After about 15 months, I thought I had been a survivor long enough to lose my identity as a cancer patient. I was on a trip in Europe with all my hair grown back and saluting myself as no person on the continent knew my history. Some people addressed me in German so I knew they were not seeing any 'survivor' label as they missed the American tourist cues.

Grounded back in USA, I returned to my survivor status. However, I rose above the feeling of being defined by cancer, a disease. Cancer is no longer a part of my identity. Cancer has no power over me.

THE VICTORY IS OURS

With all thoughts of a battle behind us, the victory over cancer is **always** ours. Cancer remains powerless and never wins as there is no battle; there is no winner nor is there a loser. We have no choice but to trust that God will carry out His plan in our lives, knowing nothing we do will change that plan. We simply must trust God to know what is best for our lives.

"He who believes in me will live, even though he dies; and whoever lives and believes in me will never die,..." John 11:26 NIV

"When Jesus was raised from the dead, it was a signal of the end of death-as-the-end." Romans 6:5-6 MSG

Would it not be a gift of grace to be spared from extreme suffering? In medical terminology, it is referred to as 'Quality of Life' issues.

"The good men perish; The godly die before their time and no one seems to care or wonder why. No one seems to realize that God is taking them away from the evil days ahead. For the godly who die shall rest in peace." Isaiah 57:1-2 TLB

This ensures us it is SAFE to believe earthly death is only the end of pain, the end of unanswered questions, and the end of hurts. Eternal life in heaven will be rewarded to faithful believers and will be pain-free.

"When this body that decays is changed into a body that cannot decay, and this mortal body is changed into a body that will live forever, then the teaching of Scripture will come true: "Death is turned into Victory!" 1 Corinthians 15:54 (God's Word)

Early after my cancer diagnosis, I started to believe God's plan for me would be surviving my first encounter with cancer. Outwardly, many people commented on my positive attitude and asked how I could be so confident of God's plan. I never knew as I trusted this would be the outcome. Delays during treatment jolted my security, but in the end, each detour strengthened my faith in the plan; I knew I would be cancer free. If I have a reoccurrence of cancer in the future, I will start over and trust the Lord again to be my guide. I have no reason to think about it now.

"Trust the Lord completely; don't ever trust yourself." Proverbs 3:5 TLB

A favorite song that was often requested during my Sunday School days was "Stand Up, Stand Up for Jesus", partly because we got to jump up from our chairs and stand up for Jesus. It was more than faith in action quite literally, it was also learning and internalizing what Jesus will do for us. My favorite line has always been "From victory unto victory….." Medical treatments can take us down long, difficult paths. Yet every small step along the way is a victory. Guided by God, our spirit takes us to the next step and we can feel grounded, safe and secure in God's promises for us.

"And the Lord will guide you continually, and satisfy you with all good things, and keep you healthy too……." Isaiah 58:11 TLB

TO CARE-GIVERS, SUPPORTERS AND CHEERLEADERS:

If you are currently a caregiver, family member, close friend supporter or a cheerleader for someone experiencing a health crisis, you will never be forgotten and will be appreciated in ways you may never know. Words cannot adequately express thanks to those who maintained support throughout the journey. Facing a health crisis alone has to be devastating without the encouragement of others. We all cope better when we know people care about us. Prayers of support can be felt and nothing feels better than to know someone is praying for you.

"He comforts us whenever we suffer. That is why whenever other people suffer, we are able to comfort them by using the same comfort we have received from God." 2 Corinthians 1:4 (God's Word)

We all have different experiences and I have shared my perspective of how vital care-givers are to someone in need. Throughout the book, I have mentioned ways support can be offered. I both depended and thrived upon support. My cheerleaders never let me down and stayed with me for the long haul. In my heart, I know every one of them is on stand-by for me and can be called upon again if I need them.

Hopefully, after reading about a perspective that may be somewhat different from your own, you also recognize there are multidimensional ways to view a health crisis. As each health condition is unique, so also each person will respond and cope in their own way. Listening is always appreciated. But remember that some questions are not for you to answer. That's not always easy, but respect whose decision it is. Always be an active listener and not an advisor. Support by affirming and allow for some venting when frustration surfaces.

"Rejoice with those who rejoice; mourn with those who mourn." Romans 12:15 NIV

Be there to celebrate each step of progress. When an illness spans a long time, it is wonderful to never feel forgotten. When I could not leave my house and had to relinquish my social life, human contact via the internet and mail were treasured times of my day. Jan faithfully sent me an e-mail almost every day that sometimes said little more than she was thinking of me and praying for my recovery. Reassurance always gave my spirit a lift and most days a joke or funny story came as a bonus.

"An anxious heart weighs a man down, but a kind word cheers him up." Proverbs 12:25 NIV

Being a caregiver is a tremendous gift to give but it can also be a burden. If you are a primary caregiver, please be good to yourself and accept the support and prayers of others who want to help you manage the enormous physical and emotional responsibilities. Seek out community and faith based resources to help sustain you and take breaks from direct care giving.

For other supporters and friends, remember the primary caregiver whose life has also dramatically changed. From diagnosis to recovery, ten months elapsed. They were the longest ten months of my husband's life. Everyone deserves a little fresh air once in awhile. If there are children in the house, it is a great gift to take them along on your outing and try to keep their lives as normal as possible. Those of us who have been ill want our families to be able to live their usual routines as much as possible. We feel the stress if their lives are upset due to our illness.

Being a caregiver is much easier if others help out. It is more than okay to ask for help even though it is very hard to do so. Two web resources are:

1. Share the Care at www.sharethecare.org. They have created a model organizing how to share care and are dedicated to educating care-giving communities about this effective model.
2. The Patient/Partner project at www.thepatientpartnerproject.org is a program focused on helping cancer patients by helping their partners. Part of their site has an open forum for participating in caregiver discussions.

"Be the change you want to see in the world." Mahatma Gandhi

All survivors have been given the gift of their personal experience. Each of us has a unique medical situation, but there is a level of understanding and a connection between survivors. Opportunities to be a caregiver will present themselves in the future and by sharing your experiences you will help other care-givers to learn how to be more effective. You need only to be willing to share.

An unhealthy body needs help to keep the spirit healthy. We need practice using God's word. Turning to God in prayer for guidance requires some discipline. It's very difficult to do this by yourself, but a fellowship of believers makes it so much easier. It goes both ways, too. As we give of ourselves to others, so much more comes back in the sharing.

I had recently completed treatment when Julie, who attended the same church as I did, started treatment for breast cancer. Our pastor had been nudging us together and we made an instant connection once we met. While I initially had hoped to be reaching out and supporting Julie, I found I was gaining far more support from her. We fully understood each other's emotions and mental turmoil/ stress over making medical choices, and could skip right to the heart of each issue. Opposite of my treatment, Julie started with chemo-therapy and had surgery later. She had to make choices and deci-sions and took the time to get a couple of opinions. With all the information gathered, it became overwhelming to decide which path to take. Together, we decided she should postpone the surgery at least a week until she could feel her spirit guide her in the right direction. It was only because Julie was exhausted from the mental stress of trying to decide what to do with the surgery that she even asked me if I thought she had the nerve to call and postpone her surgery. I supported her all the way and assured her she could both make the call and needed to do it, although I volunteered to make the call for her. In true form, she called herself.

We both prayed and she asked others to pray for the guidance she needed. Two days later, it happened. Julie felt peace and knew exactly what to do and which doctor should do it. She scheduled the surgery, all went well and she has had no regrets.

I hoped that I would have answers for Julie, giving her advice, telling her what to do because I was the experienced one. But it was never my choice nor my decision. I knew I had been guided by my spirit. In my heart, I knew she would feel guidance too, but we would have to pray for what that peace. We prayed for her spirit to guide her and give her peace of mind. Our prayers were answered the day Julie called and told me she was at peace with the plan.

Julie is the quiet type and would probably deny it, but she's my hero. The one I started out to help gave me back so much more and still does.

The following **Principles of Care-Giving** are courtesy of Pastor Robert Albers, Ph.D.

1. Care-Giving means that people will not care about how much you know until they first know how much you care.
2. Care-Giving is not so much a technique to be learned as it is an art to be cultivated.

3. Care-Giving is the art of involving one's self in another person's reality and allowing the image of God in us to respond to the reality of God in the other person.
4. Care-Giving is the art of weaving a tapestry that acknowledges the complexity of human life in its individual and corporate expressions. It must be "holistic" in its vision and understanding of ministry. (The Whole person = the body, mind and spirit)
5. Care-Giving is the art of integrating the tradition of faith with the practice of ministry and allowing our care giving to shape our understanding of faith.
6. Care-Giving is the art of developing personal sensitivity to the plurality of cultures and lifestyles in our community.
7. Care-Giving is the art of being open to the guidance of the gracious Spirit of God in order that the Spirit of God's grace might be experienced in our ministry with others.
8. Care-Giving is the art of discerning and utilizing the gifts of the members of the whole Body of Christ in order that all members of Body of Christ might be served.
9. Care-Giving is the art of allowing the questions of faith and life to be raised in an atmosphere of acceptance and love both for the sake of others as well as for ourselves.
10. Care-Giving is realizing our need for care as well as caring for the needs of others.

CARINGBRIDGE™

I highly recommend every caregiver visit the website of CaringBridge at www.caringbridge.org. It is best described by its ten-minute video at the site. It is a nonprofit organization "offering free personalized Web sites to those wishing to stay in touch with family and friends during significant life events. Our mission is to bring together a global community of care powered by the love of family and friends in an easy, accessible and private way." Families can post journal entries and photos. Visitors can leave messages in the Guestbook. As of Jan. 3, 2006, over 34,000 CaringBridge sites have been hosted, over 203 million visits to those sites and over 5 million guestbook messages. This resource is a marvelous opportunity not to miss and one to be cherished.

If you want to express to someone that you care and yet feel you do not have the words, there are many wonderful greeting cards available that you can send. The recipient still feels you have shared a little Christian love and your thoughtfulness will warm their heart. In this age of e-mails, I still enjoyed getting "real" mail from the mailbox as I could keep it to read over again and again.

PLEASE SHARE

There are countless ways to support and encourage each other. On my website, www.ahealthyspirit.info, I have a section where you can add your ideas of ways you were supported or suggestions from care-givers. The only purpose is to share. In advance, I thank you for giving these suggestions and know someone will benefit from your gift of experience and the love you share with others.

WORKS CONSULTED

Albers Ph.D., Pastor Robert. Professor of Pastoral Theology and Pastoral Care in St. Paul, MN, 2005.

Becker, Dr. Marty. The Healing Power of Pets . New York, NY: Hyperion, 2002.

Benson, MD., Herbert. Timeless Healing: The Power and Biology of Belief. New York: Fireside Books, 1996.

Berman, MD., Phillip., Founder of www.RedToeNail.org, 2005.

Centers for Disease Control and Prevention. A National Action Plan for Cancer Survivorship: Advancing Public Health Strategies. www.cdc.gov/cancer/survivorship, 2005.

Chiappone, Judie. Sacred Choices. Winter Springs, FL: Holistic Reflections, Inc., 2000.

Clifford, Christine. Not now...I'm Having a No Hair Day. Minneapolis, MN: University of Minnesota Press, 1996.

Cancer Information Group.CURE Cancer Updates, Research & Education magazine. Publication free for cancer patients and caregivers at www.curetoday.com CUREXtra is a monthly publication available on line also at www.curetoday.com

Dickey, Christopher. "Near The Edge of the Abyss." Newsweek August 15, 2005: pg. 29

Grossman Ph.D., LP, Dale Ellen. Licensed psychologist in Shoreview, MN, 2005.

A Handbook of Hope and Healing- Minnesota Breast Cancer Resource 2003-2004. Sponsored by the Susan G. Komen Breast Cancer Foundation, Minnesota Affiliate. 2003.

Lee, Betsy. The Healing Moment. Nashville, TN: Thomas Nelson, Inc., 1994.

Levin Ph.D., Jeff. God, Faith, and Health. New York, NY: John Wiley & Sons, 2001.

Lucado, Max. A Gentle Thunder. Dallas, TX: World Publishing, 1995.

Lucado, Max. In the Eye of the Storm. Dallas, TX: World Publishing, 1991.

Naparstek, Belleruth. Staying Well with Guided Imagery. New York, NY: Warner Books, 1994.

National Sleep Foundation. 2005 Sleep in America Poll. www.sleepfoundation.org pg. 7.

Nelson, Mary J. Grace for Each Hour. Bloomington, MN: Bethany House Publishers, 2005.

Richardson, Cheryl. The Unmistakable Touch of Grace. New York, NY: Free Press, 2005

Spiegel, David MD. Associate Chair of the Department of Psychiatry and Behavioral Sciences at Stanford University School of Medicine and Director of the Center on Stress and Health in Stanford, CA, 2005.

Thompson, Nathan. Senior Pastor of Shepherd of the Hills Lutheran Church in Shoreview, MN, 2004.

Umbreit, Alexa and Mark. Pathways to Spirituality and Healing. Minneapolis, MN: Fairview Press, 2002

Warren, R. Purpose Driven Life, The by RICK WARREN. Copyright 2002 by Rick Warren.

Weber, Stu. SPIRIT WARRIORS. Sisters, OR: Multnomah Publishers, 2001.

MUSIC

The Prayer. Warner Tamerlane Publishing Corp. Performed by Andrea Bocelli and Celine Dion on the "Andrea Bocelli Sogno" CD, 1998.

This is Your Gift. Garden City Music Performed by John Tesh on the John Tesh Christmas Worship CD. 2002.

INTERNET RESOUCES

ALPHA – free courses for exploring Christian beliefs at www. alphausa.com and www.alphacanada.com

American Cancer Society   www.cancer.org

Berman, MD., Phillip, Cancer blog site at www.redtoenail.org

CaringBridge – free web sites for journal entries and photos with guest books for leaving messages at www.caringbridge.org

CURE Magazine – Cancer Updates, Research and Education www.curetoday.com for quarterly publication or CUREXtra, a monthly on line publication

Guided Imagery and Affirmations:Bellaruth Naperstek's work at www.healthjourneys.com
The Academy of Guided Imagery for local practitioners at www.academyforguidedimagery.com

Lance Armstrong Foundation at www.laf.org

Look Good…Feel Better at www.lookgoodfeelbetter.org

Lotsa Helping Hands web calendar to help organize helpers at www.lotsahelpinghands.com

Love Your Neighbor support program at www.shepherdshoreview.org

Patient/Partner Project help for cancer patients by helping their partners at www.thepatientpartnerproject.org

Prayers for healing at www.prayerventures.org

Share the Care to organize a group to help give care at www.sharethecare.org

Sound Machines to aid sleep at www.marpac.com

Susan G. Komen Breast Cancer Foundation at www.komen.org

SUPPLEMENTS:

Natural Medicine Database at www.naturaldatabase.com offers reliable, up to date factual scientific data on most herbs and supplements. Cost is $90 yearly.

Cancer Nutrition at www.cancernutritioninfo.com has the most current research in an understandable format. Offers recipes and ideas for symptom management. Free trial period and then $20 per year fee.

American Institute of Cancer Research at www.aicr.org

CancerRD at www.cancerrd.com for reliable information about nutrition and cancer, recipes, menus and questions answered.

American Dietetic Association at www.eatright.org for general nutrition information.

Quackery at www.quackwatch.com reviews questionable practices.

Printed in the United States
104703LV00008B/255/A